THE SNOW PAPERS

THE
SNOW PAPERS
A Memoir of Illusion, Power-Lust, and Cocaine

BY RICHARD SMART

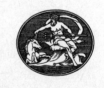

The Atlantic Monthly Press
BOSTON / NEW YORK

FIRST EDITION

LIBRARY OF CONGRESS CATALOGING-IN-PUBLICATION DATA

Smart, Richard.
  The snow papers.

  1. Smart Richard.   2. Narcotic addicts — United States
— Biography.   3. Cocaine habit — United States.   I. Title.
HV5805.S62A37   1985   362.2'93'0924   [B]   85-47996
ISBN 0-87113-030-0

BP
Published simultaneously in Canada

PRINTED IN THE UNITED STATES OF AMERICA

For my children,

Ursula, Lisa, and Geoffrey,

with a loving hope that they and their generation
will be wise enough in values, and strong enough
in will, to do things differently

Acknowledgments

I OWE a large debt of gratitude to a few people who were instrumental in the development of this book. John Seigenthaler, an old friend and colleague from Robert Kennedy's presidential campaign, thought that my story was important and needed to be told, and he armed me with a strong recommendation and introduced me to Harry Evans, editor in chief of the Atlantic Monthly Press.

Harry believed in the book, agreed to publish it, and — at a time in my life when a more cautious soul, quite understandably, might have considered me an unacceptable investment risk — provided the financial support I needed to get it written. Equally importantly, he provided much-needed moral support, and his early advice and counsel were invaluable in helping me shape my approach to the work.

Joyce Johnson has been both the most sympathetic and the toughest of editors. Her astute perceptions have clarified the substance of what I've had to say, and her gentle but rigorous discipline has greatly improved my way of saying it.

Most of all, I thank my wife, Yolaine, without whose loyalty and encouragement there would be no book at all. She has had to live through many awful events twice —

once when they happened, and again through our painful, studied recollection of them for publication to the world. For that, she has earned some kind of award as a champion of emotional stamina.

Preface

THIS book is about my search for a niche in Paradise. A place, first envisioned in my boyhood dreams, of wealth, power, prestige, and the sweet life. It is the story of how, along the way, I got blinded by a snowstorm, made a wrong turn, and began a long descent into Hell.

In its most obvious dimension this is an account of my use of cocaine to wreak devastation in my life and, more tragically, in the lives of many who are dear to me, who trusted me, and who also became victims of the drug — not through their use of it but through mine. As best I can, I've abandoned preachments. What began as a polemic on the dangers of a fashionable drug's destructive properties, and a dissertation on social forces conducive to drug abuse, became instead an effort to understand the properties of my *own being* that, when mixed with cocaine, produced a synergism of evil.

An understanding of myself required that I reopen years that had long since been locked up and put away. I did not have the help of professional therapy in my fight against cocaine abuse, the most obvious symptom of my illness (and make no mistake, drug abuse is *not* the illness, only the most awful symptom of a deeper pathology). Nor are the memories and thoughts that I've put down here the products of psychoanalysis. I took the journey into my past alone; so I anticipate that some good psychoanalysts may find my unguided introspection incomplete and maybe, in some respects, simply wrongheaded. Yet, regardless of such possible missteps, I know that this venture of self-discovery has given me a handle on who I am and why I've done what I have, and therefore a handle on reality. To get a firm grip on reality, and to hold on tight despite the pain of a very rough ride, is the nonnegotiable price of the journey to health. And to retrieved honor.

I cannot prove that my discoveries about myself give a broadly true answer to the question of why certain personalities, who are otherwise successful in their lives' external aspects, are especially vulnerable to cocaine's murderous potential. But I deeply believe it to be so. For those who have already surrendered themselves to entrapment, and for those sorely tempted to pursue a drug-induced respite from reality, I hope that my description of myself and my life will give them a shock of self-recognition that will promote healing in the one case and preventive treatment in the other.

This story does not present a rounded view of my life and attitudes. I have intentionally emphasized aspects that I believe contributed most directly to the large mistakes. Seen whole, my childhood, my relations with my family, my first marriage, my inner life of the mind, were neither joyless nor bereft of positive attitudes. There was much that was good and rewarding. But, given this work's purpose, a life picture that emphasizes the shadows and mutes the light is both unavoidable and useful. This is the story of what went wrong with my life, not what went right with it. There is no need to elaborate here on my present feelings about drugs; the story itself is clear on that. But the book really is about diseased values that contribute to cocaine addiction and other destructions, and, as to that subject, I feel compelled to make a prefatory statement:

These are attitudes toward the world that I no longer hold.

This is a work of nonfiction. In an effort to spare embarrassment to people I have written about who have used drugs, I have disguised their identities. I have also disguised the identities of some other people who have not used drugs where their identification might reveal the identity of the drug users.

For the public, I hope my narrative will provide a useful object lesson. But to my wife, Yolaine, who suffered so much yet kept her faith and strength while encouraging, cajoling, and sometimes intimidating me toward survival, I offer the book not as a compendium of horrors that she knows all too well, but as a love story. Told at last without mirrors and illusions.

Shenandoah Valley Farm
McGaheysville, Virginia
February 1985

Contents

THE SNOW PAPERS

1
Glimpse of Paradise

MIDMORNING of a Sunday in the summer of 1976 the telephone rang in my San Francisco bachelor apartment, arousing me from a deep recuperative sleep mandated by the sybaritic frolics of the night before. The familiar voice of Nina — she and her international investment banker husband, Mel, were among my oldest and dearest friends — cut through my fogginess to invite me to the finals of a tennis tournament that afternoon at the Cow Palace. I mumbled, "Thank you but no thank you," explaining that last night's festivities had been brutally long.

Nina conveyed sympathy for my debilitation but wouldn't be put off. The match was going to be great, and she and Mel wanted very much to see me after much too long a time. Besides, they wanted to meet the new young lady I was seeing, who, she added with a sharp needle, was rumored to be a distinct improvement over my other recent companions. And, as for my crippled condition, "Don't worry about that," she said. "Mel and I have just the thing to give you and your little girlfriend a quick pick-me-up." Knowing Nina, I concluded that it would be less exhausting to go than to argue the point, advised Melanie, who lay beside me in an equally wasted state, of our afternoon plans, draped my arm across the small of her back, set the alarm, and dropped off for two more hours of precious sleep.

Melanie had virtually presented herself to me on a silver platter, a lovely gift that came, somewhat miraculously, just when I needed it. I had been separated from my wife of sixteen years for nearly a year. It had been an easy separation. Arlene and I had simply grown apart, year by year, in increasingly diverging directions until no points of meaningful emotional contact were left. We both were saddened and our two girls were deeply hurt, but there were no animosities, and affections remained. Every couple of weeks I would return to the house for dinner with the family and watch a little television, occasions that were sentimental punctuation marks in my new separate life.

I had looked forward to my singleness with relish. The consulting business I had formed several years earlier was prospering, and my reputation as an astute policy analyst and lobbyist/lawyer had also blossomed. I owned a condominium at Lake Tahoe and vacationed in Hawaii.

With the tension of a failed marriage put behind me, I could concentrate on securing and expanding my newly won power and take the careful steps that would turn it into wealth. And, freed from the need to maintain even the appearances of fidelity, I could now openly pursue my long-standing and compelling avocation — women. I took a studio apartment high up in one of the Golden Gateway Center towers, the city's most fashionable downtown address; filled it with ferns, palms, and grape ivy; bought a huge multicolored candle in the shape of half a watermelon and hung it from the ceiling with braided leather strings; filled my record cabinet with Vivaldi and Joan Baez; and acquired a king-sized water bed that I covered with a custom-made patchwork quilt filled with eiderdown. There, with a vast view of the bay stretching out below, I created

4

the quintessential rich, hip San Francisco love nest of the seventies.

The part of my plan that pertained to business went well; the part that pertained to women did not. A week out of my family house, I climbed into my water bed with a woman I had wanted for months and for the first time learned the shock of impotence. We had an intense emotional involvement with each other and wanted desperately to share our bodies. But that first humiliating failure assured my mind that others would follow, and my fear became a self-fulfilling prophecy. For months we thrashed about, our lust exhausting itself not in copulation, but in frustration, tears, and rage. We decided that a change of place might help, but it didn't work any better on the floor than in bed. And even a week together in the primal air of the Yucatán wilds failed to produce a cure. The lady finally couldn't take it anymore, we abandoned the challenge, and I decided it was time for some psychoanalysis.

After four months of it, I was functioning heroically again. It was unclear whether credit belonged to the doctor; to the passage of time after a marital breakup that may have been more traumatic for me than I knew; or to the tender ministrations of the blond, middle-aged divorcée from the suburbs whom I met at Perry's, San Francisco's premier watering hole and body exchange for horny young professionals and business people.

I should have been elated with my recovery; my nights could again be as rewarding as my days at the office. But a new unhappiness replaced the one I had overcome. One evening, halfway through a bottle of Jack Daniels, I realized that never before in my entire life had I lived alone. In college and law school there had been roommates, in the army there had been other soldiers in the barracks, and all the rest of my life I had had the company of either parents or a wife and children, or an occasional girlfriend to assure me daily of my worth. Even during my monthly business trips to Washington, I had managed to keep my bed at the Madison occupied by one or another local friend. The truth was, I couldn't bear being alone for even a single night.

I had always been a compulsive pursuer of women, but in the past the interstices of my marriage had been selectively filled by the relatively few who attracted me with their beauty, intelligence, sensuality, and established positions in my world. Women who, I convinced myself, were engaged with me in "meaningful" relationships, however occasional or brief. But now it was different. I had no time for either selectivity or protracted seduction; the bed must be kept occupied. So for months there had been almost nightly forays into the city's hottest bars in search of conquests. Sometimes they came with me for a night, sometimes for three or four, and, despite my unease, one relationship lasted for two weeks. They went in and out of my apartment like holiday shoppers through a revolving door.

However exciting the nights, they always were followed by bleak mornings. Who *was* this person and why was she here? She could screw all right, but could she talk? I couldn't remember much conversation. How did I say good-bye? "Well, we better hurry out of here, I have to run to the office, I'll call you tomorrow," knowing full well I wouldn't. They didn't care about me any more than I cared about them. With growing agitation, I began to ask myself where the woman of quality was, the woman whose conversation, laughter, and intensely sincere body would polish up my self-esteem and give me a private relationship to match my public image.

That was a question that others were asking as well. If my much-anticipated bachelorhood had become a nightmare for me, it had become something of a joke to my closest friends. This was a sophisticated group — Mel the international banker, James the corporate lawyer, and Michael the millionaire investor — and they had expected much more of me. They kidded me mercilessly about the assortment of dicey women I was seen with, but the humor was leavened with real concern. They sensed my loneliness and hoped I would at least find someone who might give me some transient joy; someone attractive enough to join us in our dinners at the city's elegant restaurants, who could speak in compound sentences and select the proper fork. We were a snobby little group, and the standards for admission to it were very high.

James's wife, Catherine, who had always felt herself responsible for my welfare, gratuitously undertook a talent search on my behalf. One day she telephoned me at the office in a state of great excitement. "Richard, I know somebody who's dying to go out with you, a brilliant girl who's getting her MBA at Stanford. Her name is Melanie Andrews and you simply must give her a call."

And that's exactly what I did. Melanie Andrews gave a little gasp of embarrassment, recovered quickly, and said, "Well, I don't know that I'm exactly *dying* to go out with you, but yes, I do think it would be quite nice."

We met that evening for a get-acquainted drink. I told her that I was leaving the next day for a weekend at Lake Tahoe and asked if she would like to go along. Without even a pretense of thoughtful consideration, she immediately said that she would love to. We arrived at the lake at three the following afternoon, carried our suitcases in, and, without unpacking, jumped forthrightly into bed. I was amazed. This was a very classy girl, yet it had been so free and easy, the mutual expectation of immediate sex tacitly understood. Well, it was 1976 in California after all, the middle of the first decade of the new morality. A time and place when even nice girls, if they had the urge, would do it quickly and eagerly and without a twinge of guilt. Times had changed, and my own repressed youth seemed light-years away.

7

Melanie was the perfect symbol of the good life that was blossoming for me in 1976. She was a very bright young woman, as gifted in animated conversation as she was in bed. Slender, rounded and firm in buttocks and breasts, five and a half feet tall with rich black hair that fell softly to the middle of her shoulder blades, and possessed of an innocent yet wild face, she announced to me and the world my prosperity, success, charm, and desirability. I was forty-four and she was twenty-two, which was of course just perfect. It wasn't a relationship that would be forever, but for the time being it certainly would do.

San Francisco in 1976, with my lush bachelor apartment, water bed, condominium, and Melanie, was a long distance from Provo, Utah, in 1932. It was nearly half a century since I had been born in that pious place without gleaming skyscrapers, fashionable boutiques, or elegant French restaurants. Nestled up against the foothills of the Wasatch Mountains and surrounded by small farms eked out of the desert, Provo was a tiny oasis of lawns and trees that probably had no more than two or three thousand people then, including a few hundred students at the Brigham Young Academy. The residents lived in small square houses made of brick or stucco; did their dancing Saturday nights in the church recreation hall; bought their denim overalls and boots, and their Sunday go-to-meetin' suits and print dresses, either at Montgomery Ward's or the little church-owned store; and, when they could manage it during the terrible Depression years, celebrated holidays with pot roast cooked deep brown all the way through, mashed potatoes with heavy brown gravy, and vegetables that the family had picked in the summer and the women had canned and stored in their cellars. Folks hadn't heard of "cuisine"; instead they praised "a good solid meal that will stick to your ribs through the winter." Cholesterol hadn't been discovered yet, and parents insisted to their children that the best part of the meat was the gristle and fat. Everybody drank mineral-hard water that came out of the ground; nobody had heard of Perrier.

Along with much of the world, Provo has changed a lot since I was born there on Columbus Day, 1932. Now a thriving city, it has prosperous shops featuring the latest fashions, the tiny academy has grown into Brigham Young University, the world's largest church-owned school, and the plateaus and foothills to the north and east are filled with expensive ranch-style houses, some with pools and tennis courts. In his book *The Executioner's Song*, Norman Mailer made Provo famous as the spawning ground of Gary Gilmore, one of the less repellent multiple murderers of our time. Fame came to Provo again when the university's football team won a national championship, and the town became infected with a dose of hubris.

But even though blessed by prosperity, touched by murder, and crazed by football mania, Provo's business remains essentially what it always has been — religion. Only forty miles south of Salt Lake City, the spiritual and banking capital of the Church of Jesus Christ of Latter-Day Saints, Provo is the Mormons' academic center — the place where mathematics, economics, literature, and marketing are now taught side-by-side with the revealed word of the Lord. With all the new sophistications, three constants remain — piety, a revered pioneer heritage, and belief in a direct pipeline to the living God.

In 1932 the town was only one short generation removed from a hard-scrabble western settlement created to serve the needs of farmers, ranchers, and miners struggling to extract a living from the salty, arid land of Utah. The couples who were raising families in Utah that year — my parents among them — were themselves the grandchildren, and in some cases the *children*, of pioneers who, in the mid-nineteenth century, had crossed a continent, to settle the West.

My paternal great-grandfather, a giant of a man with a massive black beard, was the biggest sheep rancher in the Utah Territory. His son, William, was a slight, sickly man but as tough and harsh as a nail. On the order of the church's Prophet, my grandfather set out on horseback and led the settlement of the Uintah Basin, a vast desert valley in eastern Utah populated by sagebrush, jackrabbits, coyotes, rattlesnakes, and hostile Indians. There, he founded towns and, tolerating weakness in neither himself nor his followers, invoked the Word of the Lord. He taught his son — my father — the evils of tobacco and liquor with the business end of a horsewhip. Grandfather Smart died when I was a small boy, but I remember something of him. He had a thin, chalk-white face, and he wore a black suit with a black tie under a wing collar. He was starkly bald from some illness, and through a pair of round, rimless glasses there pierced the searing, inescapable eyes of an Abraham. Grandmother — portly, warm, and loving — was his antithesis. I don't know what his other women were like; by then, polygamy had long since been outlawed, as a condition of Utah's statehood, and, in loyalty and righteousness, Grandfather had secreted his other wives away in dispersed, safe places.

In his piety, Dad was his father's son, although he taught righteousness to my three sisters and two brothers and me not with the horsewhip that his father had favored, but with his own quiet, gentle example and dry humor. He devoted his life to the pursuit of exaltation in the Kingdom of God. We had followed him from Provo to Reno and then to Portland, Oregon, as he answered the call of the church to move to new places to sell life insurance for the church-owned company.

For many years, I tried to follow Dad's teachings, but,

with adolescence finished, the adult world opened up before me and I opted for the pleasures to be had in this life in lieu of the vague glories promised for the next. My opulent life in San Francisco was a distinct improvement over the satisfactions of the spirit to be had from adherence to Puritan disciplines. Melanie's flesh was infinitely more warming than a bishop's sermon. And, with overcooked roast beef a faint memory from a distant childhood, my palate had become comfortably attuned to caviar, medallions of veal in lemon butter sauce, and the best wines.

By 1976, the dry Utah desert, and the religion and lifestyle it symbolized, were far behind me. I was at the height of my powers — not quite rich yet, but getting there; and living the sweet life. To spend a pleasant Sunday afternoon watching a tennis match with my young lover was a fitting thing.

With the ring of the alarm clock, I roused Melanie and told her we had to get moving. She rolled herself into a ball, and pulled the quilt over her head. "Come on," I said. "I feel as awful as you do, but I promised Nina we'd go and there will be some good tennis to watch. Besides, she said that they had something that would give our crippled bodies a real pickup, whatever that means."

"Okay, I'll go," she said, "even if I do feel just terrible. But if she thinks she's going to pop a couple of uppers down my throat, she can forget it. I've had amphetamines once or twice studying for exams, but anything like that today would crack my nerves in half and send me through the roof."

It was a fast-tempoed match at the Cow Palace but I soon dozed off in Mel's box. I was next conscious that he was shaking me by the shoulder, his face up close to mine. In a mildly conspiratorial tone, he said, "Hey, Richard, come with me to the bathroom." I responded with something like, "Mel, that's very weird. Women go to the bathroom together to gossip and put on their makeup. Men don't; and even if they did, I'm too exhausted to move an inch."

Again, insistence. "Come on, Richard. I'm going to give you a treat that will make you feel fantastic." A sigh of resignation, and off I shuffled. The first of hundreds of such trips that I would take over the next seven years — not to relieve myself, but to feel "fantastic."

This Sunday, which now seems so long ago, was the day of my initiation into a world within a world, in which the ritual "trip to the bathroom" was but the first of a number of bizarre customs that ultimately were to become integrated into my daily life.

As the line shortened, and Mel and I approached our respective turns in the privacy of the WC, my friend whispered to me that he had a bottle of snow and asked whether I had ever tried it.

"Snow?" I said. "Mel, what the hell are you talking about?"

"You know, coke — cocaine."

Learning that I was an innocent, he explained that he would go in first and have a couple of "toots." He would then emerge and discreetly slip me the bottle. There was a tiny spoon attached to the lid that was to be filled with the powder, which was then to be inhaled into each nostril. I was to replace the lid carefully and emerge — without looking guilty — from the stall. Above all, I was not to spill any of the powder, because it was *very* expensive.

I followed Mel's instructions to the letter. I told him, "Thank you, it's been very interesting to sniff powder up my nose, but so what?" He just smiled gently and we returned to our seats, whereupon Nina escorted Melanie to the powder room, where the ladies were to repeat the ritual.

I was still exhausted and prepared to doze off again, the lobs, smashes, and volleys notwithstanding. But, after a few moments slumped in my seat, a truly wondrous thing occurred. I was awake! Not *just* awake, but *marvelously* awake. The arena suddenly was filled with a brighter, energizing light, the yellow tennis ball danced across the net with a new liveliness, and I was aware of myself actually entranced by its spinning seams. A match that had been a bore to my earlier exhausted self had become a thing of beauty, and the four of us were now immersed in its every nuance. We were no longer merely passive spectators — let alone sleepy ones. We were *participants* — unbelievably alive and happy. Our comments about the match became absolutely trenchant. I had never been so alert or so brilliant and witty in conversation. In all my life, I had never felt so sure of myself. Or so powerful.

After the match we all dined at a North Beach restaurant, talking brilliantly through the night and into the next morning, saying farewell only as the light of the Monday sun began to glow over the hills to the east. Melanie and I returned to my apartment, where — after another couple of snorts of cocaine left with us by the ever-generous Mel — we made a new and remarkably exciting kind of love.

Even now, nine long years later, my mind's eye reproduces that tennis match and the night that followed with absolute clarity. The images that come to me are so real, it all could have happened yesterday. If emotional milestones are what we tend to remember, this — my day of tennis and cocaine — was a milestone indeed. On a balmy afternoon in San Francisco in the summer of 1976, in the innocent milieu of a tennis tournament, the seeds were sown. Loving friends. A couple of snorts of glistening white powder. Profound new understandings. A surpassing euphoria.

I was nearing the top of my world in that summer of 1976, relishing the rewards of a trek that had begun a decade earlier, fueled by the excitement and visions of the wonderful sixties. A trek toward money, glamour, voluptuous pleasures, and a large dose of power. And now, through the generous spirit of a good friend, I had a new drug that multiplied the pleasures and cast the visions in a brilliant new light. If the seventies were the time for the fullest enjoyment of life's bounties, it was in the sixties that my appetite for them had been whetted and refined. The only surprise was that my initiation into the cocaine-snorting rituals of the liberal elite had taken so long.

2
The Sixties

IN 1960, I was twenty-seven years old and in my last year of law school, only three years removed from Brigham Young University — the citadel of old Mormon virtues where I had lived out the last chapter of that part of my life which had been indentured to parental dictates. Among the country's law schools, Yale was the fountainhead of liberal social theory and jurisprudence — the place where I learned that values were relative, not absolute; that our revered legal system was shaped by economic interests, not immutable moral principles; that America, like other countries, had been invented by self-seeking pragmatists rather than by God as a shelter for His Chosen People.

At Yale I learned that a revolution was in the making; and at Yale I picked up the credentials that could put me in the front ranks of the intellectual elite that would lead it. The difference between BYU and Yale was like the difference between night and day. For me, BYU had represented an obsolete world of repressive religious autocracy that had troubled me since childhood, a world to which I had felt compelled to pay homage despite my disbelief, and from which I had been afraid to escape despite my anxiety. The sudden move from BYU to Yale was like walking out of a shadow into liberating sunlight; at last I could see myself as an autonomous being, and I knew who I was.

I felt more than a release from Mormonism's theological shackles. I felt freed from old-fashioned thinking about the nature and meaning of American life. In its insistence that America was literally God's country, and that traditional American values were expressions of God's will, the Mormon Church had functioned as a self-appointed guardian of capitalism, virginity, white supremacy, and the lives of unborn children more than a century before the Moral Majority was even a gleam in Jerry Falwell's eye. The church had been not only the Protector of the Faith but, by powerful indirection, the arbiter of my family's political devotions and private morality as well. So, with my new freedom from what I saw as an absolutist religion, I also felt liberated from efforts to control my political thoughts and suppress my instinct for moral experiments.

A whole new ball game with vague and flexible rules was shaping up; my father and his generation of Mormon bishops and other American Philistines had grown too old to be taken seriously as either players or referees. Unfettered from old strictures, a new generation would try this, then try that, and judge its own performance — not against some old dogma, but against the test of what made us feel free, enlightened, and good. We'd make up any necessary rules as we went along.

I had been on the tag end of what contemporary historians prematurely called the silent generation of the fifties. By the 1960s, our task was to find ourselves a good place to ride on the true wave of the future. Not the big, roiling, noisy wave that the kids were riding; that one was making the stalwarts of respectability nervous and, like all towering waves, its fate would be to crash and break up on the shoals of reality, strewing its riders on the shore in wreckage. Our wave would be the calmer one, coming in behind the big breaker and born of its spirit, but flowing in with a subtler power and pushing before it the flotsam from which the new society would be built.

We didn't plant bombs, take to the streets with picket signs, or even take the more benign route of protest that led to a beatific life in a commune. We were too old for that sort of thing; we were members of a privileged, highly educated class of young professionals, well on our way toward successful and influential careers, and outraged extremism was not our style. Besides, while we knew that the rebels were pricking the country's conscience in the right places, and while we were titillated by the new morality they promised, we also knew that the new society that would emerge from the confrontation, although profoundly different from the old one, would be considerably less revolutionary than the benign state of anarchy prophesied by the rejectionist young.

Recently graduated from the best universities, employed by the best law firms or embarked on fledgling entrepreneurial ventures, and full of righteous energy coupled with astutely directed ambition, we had little taste for the kinds of confrontation that could jeopardize promising careers. But we were idealistic and highly politicized, sensitive to the winds of change that were blowing across the land, and we didn't want to end up on the wrong end of history. In short, we wanted to have life both ways — safe and adventurous. So we joined the ranks of what Tom Wolfe would brilliantly label the radical chic, working competently in our mainstream professions to secure money and power among a responsible elite, while playing at the rhetoric of social revolution and indulging in the afterhours entertainments of the wholeheartedly rebellious young.

The Robert Kennedy and Eugene McCarthy campaigns were the political vehicles of our crusade. But the flower children and radical activists instructed us upwardly mobile young liberals in much more than just the need for social and political change. They also taught us the liberating virtues of the "New Morality." I had long since discovered the clandestine pleasures to be had from challenging God's unreasonably restrictive injunction against adultery, but the afterflushes of such merriments invariably had been sullied by guilt. Now an entire generation rose up to declare that my sexual pathology was not only not *dirty*, but could be absolutely *virtuous;* the only requirement for philosophical purity was that, if one was going to screw indiscriminately, it had to be with the *right frame of mind.*

Marijuana was a great help in achieving "the right frame of mind," as well as a wonderful pleasure. Father had taught us children that pleasure and joy were the fruits of hard work and solemn prayer and that gratification lay at the end of a long road of pious industry. Well, Dad's generation knew nothing of pot; it brought peace and pleasure, and freedom from the burden of responsibility, in a couple of minutes — and without any work at all. Pot made the whole world seem benign. When under its spell, I bore my enemies no malice; in fact I *had* no enemies. Evil ceased to exist, and because there was no evil, there was no guilt.

Everything was *good* — especially the bodies of women. The sensuality of their touch, magnified a thousand times by the herb, reduced old commandments to absurd anachronisms. A new age of revelation was upon me, and the revelation was *feeling.* The Word was dead, suffocated by the rush of ineffable cellular communication, to be had everywhere about me simply for the asking. When I smoked marijuana, my past, full of stern injunctions and judgmental ghosts, vanished in a puff of pungent smoke; and the present exposed its purified self, stripped of antilife shadows of demanding creditors and cloistering wives, there for the taking in all its hedonistic splendor.

I would leave idealism and my youth in the sixties. But I didn't depart that wonderful decade bereft of baggage. I had a new view of life. My years of agonizing ambivalence about the old virtues taught by my parents and the church of my childhood were behind me. In their stead, I carried solemn new understandings and delightful new habits.

The new life that was born at Yale Law School and blossomed in the sixties in Wall Street law practice, and then in the rarefied air of San Francisco affluence, was far removed in miles and mind from the one I had lived before. Mental adventures replaced rote recitations of religious Articles of Faith. Black-tie political fund-raisers in elegant hotels, at a thousand dollars a head, replaced church picnics and tacky dances in church recreation halls. An active social conscience replaced benign prayer, sensuality replaced moral austerity, and the immediate excitements of this world replaced the formless promises of solemn priests about the godly one to come. In New York and San Francisco and Washington, D.C., heady wines fermented, bubbling with high culture, wealth, glamour, and the excitement of a social and moral revolution, and I drank deeply. Provo, Utah, and Portland, Oregon — my early experiences in the pious provinces — became harmless memories from a world suddenly obsolete.

It was clear to me now that my salvation did not lie in some biblical heaven, but in fruition of the ultimate experience of flesh and mind. I still believed in God, but not my forefathers' God, not that fearful patriarch who rewarded piety with eternal life and punished sin with damnation. Rather, God was a happy life force, beautiful in the elusiveness of His definition and in the benignity of His will. It was comforting to continue to believe in God's vague and undemanding presence, and convenient to finally know that the passing of judgments was not His business.

If you were young, bright, ambitious, and idealistic, the last half of the decade was the headiest of times. With the streets full of demonstrations against war and Johnson, the black militants and the students redefining the structure of political power, and with a generation of rebellious young people proclaiming a new creed of sexual openness and "consciousness expansion," the Old Order — with its definitions of public and private virtue — was crumbling. Those of us who were in our thirties then — old enough to understand how the "system" worked yet young enough to be turned on by our juniors' strange mix of political idealism and unabashed hedonism — were there to pick up the pieces. As the responsible "elders" of a young generation of rebels, we would employ our expertise and ambition to fashion a new America out of the social rubble of the old one. Ours would be a country of tough, reformist politics leavened with romantic idealism and congenial to the pursuit of pleasure. We would be both the governors of this new society and the most ardent practitioners of its privileges.

By 1968, all we were waiting for was for Robert Kennedy to pick up the banner of his martyred brother and lead us. The call to arms came in the early spring. Kennedy had bided his time while Eugene McCarthy, the arrogant, quixotic, and coolly intellectual senator from Minnesota, challenged Johnson in a couple of early Democratic primaries on the single issue of the Vietnam war. With very little money, but supported by thousands of hardworking students enlisted in his "children's crusade" for peace, whose idealism was surpassed only by their political naïveté, McCarthy soundly beat Johnson in the New Hampshire primary. For President Johnson, the handwriting was on the wall.

Having successfully used McCarthy as a stalking horse to prove Johnson's vulnerability before committing himself to political risk, Kennedy summoned the press to the same Senate room where JFK had announced his candidacy eight years earlier; there he dramatically laid claim to his brother's political legacy, and told the country that he was running for President. An embittered Johnson announced that he wouldn't run for reelection.

Along with hundreds of my like-minded peers across the country, I foresaw the Kennedy renaissance as my great chance. Quite apart from the noble achievements and personal glory that a Kennedy victory would hold for me, there would be the incomparable excitement of the campaign game itself — the infinite energy, emotional intensity, and feeling of sustained power that infuses those occasional American political campaigns that are led by truly charismatic contenders. And this campaign would be a classic. On one side, the austere, Augustan McCarthy, self-enamored with belief in his own omniscience, full of bitter contempt toward Kennedy for his belated entry into the contest. And on the other side, a man driven by a different, but equally compelling, arrogance — a conviction that, by birthright, he was not only entitled to the presidency, but, through some mystical contract that bound the Kennedy family and the people together in a historic common destiny, was dutybound to capture it. Robert Kennedy's most obvious campaign weapon would be his chemistry with crowds. When, with a loose athleticism, he mounted a stage or the top of a car, his long hair disheveled by the wind, his smile flashing, there flowed between Kennedy and the assembled masses an almost palpable sensuality, a communication that was physical without touching. And when his nasal voice with its flat Boston accent spoke its impassioned rhetoric, the sharply clipped words of political exhortation merged with the beckoning body language to summon up in those who listened the belief that Robert Kennedy's historic obligation was also theirs.

But Kennedy's gift for crowd seduction was only the most public of his political armaments. Backing up the public persona, with its aura of taut passion, was the most talented bunch of political thinkers and advisers that any nonincumbent had ever taken into a political campaign, an army of politically ambitious intellectuals temporarily dispossessed of their dreams by Lee Harvey Oswald's bullets, waiting like a government in exile for the inevitable Kennedy restoration. And finally there were the operatives, a cadre of political professionals who had sharpened their teeth in the rough-and-tumble politics of Boston's Irish wards and polished them in JFK's juggernaut run for the presidency; a seasoned bunch of toughs, expert in screwing together the nuts and bolts of a campaign and greasing the machine when it squeaked — old pols with politics in their blood, soon to be in command of a nationwide apparatus of very young and very tough lawyers, hard-bitten newsmen, and other "amateurs" on leave from their jobs.

It would be the most efficient political operation that money could buy, directed from the top by the inner circle of the Kennedy clan, Robert himself, brother Ted, brother-in-law Steve Smith, and a cousin or two, all thoroughly schooled in the cardinal rule of life according to old Joe Kennedy: *Don't lose*. It would be a campaign to which the family would bring all of its assets — money, charm, zeal, limitless energy, absolute belief in their entitlement to the prize, and the ruthlessness of a gang of street fighters.

The day after Kennedy announced his candidacy, I telephoned Adam Walinsky in the senator's office in Washington. When I had arrived at Yale Law School eleven years earlier, by way of the far-flung provinces of the West, Adam had been one of my first confrontations with a new and strange species — the aggressive, abrasive, and unabashedly brilliant New York Jew.

We had become friends of sorts at Yale, playing with each other intellectually but keeping a short distance apart, like two bear cubs from different mountains put into a cage together. But with all the growing understanding, he remained a nemesis. I worked my ass off each year to keep in the top ten percent of the class, and gave myself some credit for brilliance in the achievement. Adam, with his photographic memory, read an entire page of complicated legal text at a glance, flipping through the books for maybe an hour, then spent four or five hours a day playing bridge in the student lounge. With all my hard work, he arrogantly finished each year a couple of places ahead of me in the class rankings without even seeming to try.

I could have lived with the indignity of his easy brilliance had that been all I had to contend with. But one day in our last year, after having just purchased an expensive gray tweed sports jacket at J. Press, I sat down next to him in the law library. "Dick," he said, "for some time I've been meaning to tell you something about your clothes. You wear gray a lot. You have a neutral complexion [I knew he meant "bland"], and you should never wear medium gray. It makes you look sickly. You should only wear colors that are very light or very dark. That jacket isn't at all right for you."

As in all things, his tone was certain. Even if he was wrong, how do you respond to that kind of gratuitous criticism — "Adam, you're full of shit"? Besides, despite the arrogance, he was really trying to be helpful and he wasn't wrong. I've never worn medium gray since.

That was Adam in law school. I had figured he would return to New York, become a quick star as a trial lawyer in a midtown Jewish law firm, get rich and make noise. But if I had amorphous dreams of political power in high places, Adam had *plans*, carefully laid, kept private, and, after graduation, pursued with rigor and discipline. With Robert Kennedy's election to the Senate, Adam became his chief legislative aide and speechwriter. As the fateful election of 1968 approached, he and Peter Edelman were the premier advisers who formulated Kennedy's legislative positions in the Senate. If I wanted to get into the campaign on the ground floor, Walinsky was the logical entree.

Several months before Kennedy's announcement, I had made my preliminary, carefully casual overture. During a business trip to Washington, I had invited Walinsky to lunch. We met in Kennedy's office, where Adam introduced me to the small, wiry man, the embodiment of a royalist myth already in the making, the man millions of Americans hoped would lead them back into the unfinished glories of Camelot. We exchanged pleasantries for three or four minutes. Nothing momentous was said, but, up close, the man to whose future I had mentally attached my own instantly took possession of me. He was jacketless that day, with sleeves rolled up to expose forearms with outsized muscles, collar unbuttoned, and tie pulled loose; his small eyes would pierce me, then dart restlessly about. Somehow he managed to be both with you and in a hundred other places of the mind; every word, however inconsequential in content, seemed warmed with a smoldering fire. If my decision to tie myself to Kennedy's star had initially been ninety percent mental calculation as to where my own future interests lay, this first brief meeting worked an immediate transformation. Now he had hold of my heart.

Adam and I had lunch at the Monocle, a couple of blocks from the Capitol. There were half-a-dozen enthusiastic hellos for Adam as we walked in. I noticed that Adam had changed, now that he had become Machiavelli to the heir apparent. He still had the razor-sharp mind and freely displayed it. But his caustic manner had mellowed into an almost patrician demeanor. With his rich blue pinstripe suit and muted silk tie, perfectly manicured nails, and calm, considerate manner, it was easy to imagine him as the coming generation's Clark Clifford, dispensing fifty years' worth of charm, grace, and political wisdom across Washington's establishment landscape; a public man for all seasons. Part of the change could no doubt be attributed to greater maturity; presumably all of us had grown up a little bit since graduation. But there was more to it than that. If you were in your early thirties and, in a little more than a year, expected to be either the attorney general of the United States or special counsel to the President, you could afford a little serenity to leaven the ambition. And my old friend Adam was nothing that day if not serene.

We chatted awhile about our classmates and what had become of them, told a few stories and reminisced. Over coffee, with a studied offhandedness, I asked whether he thought Kennedy would challenge Johnson for the nomination. He played the game as casually as I and said, "It's really much too early to tell. Certainly Bob's not talking about it. Johnson's looking weak right now, but he'll probably bounce back. It would take a lot of guts for somebody to challenge him from within the party. All Kennedy's thinking about right now is being a good senator from New York."

If I believed that, I could believe in the tooth fairy. But I admired Adam's coolness and his discreet loyalty to the party line of diffidence that putative candidates usually put out before their formal declarations. There was, nonetheless, the small playful smile at the end of the brief statement, and the level gaze, as he waited, over a long and very pregnant silence, to hear my response. He knew perfectly well what I was up to; nearly seven years without a word and now, just as the waters of presidential politics were starting to boil, a casual call for a pointless lunch at the Monocle? Not quite.

"Well," I said, "I'm sure that all makes sense at the moment. But if the perception changes — if he does decide to run — I want you to know that I'm for him and I want to help out in the campaign. The demands of my consulting practice are very heavy of course; but I'll make some sacrifices to do whatever I can."

"Of course," he said. "I'm glad to know of your support."

And there it was — on the table. The entire discussion of presidential politics had lasted no more than three minutes, but it was enough. I had effectively — and without seeming too hungry — implemented the cardinal rule of the ambitious political job-seeker: Get your support on record *early*. And "early" meant, at the very least, before the candidate had achieved his first big primary election victory. Better yet was to declare your affections even before your man announced his candidacy, thus proving you were a *risk-taking* opportunist, an up-front True Believer. I knew that my offhand overture had achieved its purpose. Adam would remember. If Kennedy declared, I would be in the campaign. Not at the very pinnacle; but at the top of the second tier. And after the election, that would be good enough to take me where I wanted to go in Washington.

And Walinsky did remember. When Kennedy declared his candidacy about half a year later and I telephoned Adam from San Francisco, he took the call immediately. I told him I was excited by the news and ready to go to work, and that I had mailed to him that morning a memorandum suggesting a role I could usefully perform in the California primary campaign. He said he was delighted to hear from me and would have called me anyway; they wanted me in the campaign but weren't quite sure where. Things were hectic in the office and he couldn't talk to me in detail, but somebody would get back to me in a couple of days. I could count on it.

Well I sure as hell hoped so. Adam had sounded genuinely enthusiastic, my adrenaline was flowing, and I could almost taste the sweetness of that seductive fruit which, in my fantasies, I had lusted after for so many years — power and fame in the big leagues of national politics. Yet, as my spirits soared, my lifelong anxiety, always brooding just below the surface, raised its ugly head. Why had Adam, despite his warmth, had to get off the phone so quickly? Was it just a polite kiss-off? People like me obviously were jamming Kennedy's switchboard with calls from all across the country, clamoring with their self-proclaimed brilliance and skills to get aboard the campaign. What made me think I had a special ticket?

I was thirty-five years old, but the essence of the fear was no different from that which had nearly crippled me with anxiety as a kid, waiting to hear whether I had made the football team or had been voted into an exclusive school club, or whether a desirable girl would accept my invitation to the prom. As so often had happened in my life, people had accepted my talents at face value and I had positioned myself for a large success; but, full of self-doubts that belied the confident façade, I couldn't believe — not *really* believe — that others recognized me as authentic. The next few days were hell. I was a lawyer, a financial success, a respected professional, a grown man with a wife and two daughters; yet, with all of that, I was suddenly as paralyzed as a catatonic child. I couldn't function at all in the face of even a dollop of ambiguity. For four days I sat at my desk, feigning work while doodling with a pencil and waiting for the telephone to ring, my brain alternating between fantasies of power and dark scenarios in which I was ignored and simply left behind. For four days I did nothing but dream and brood.

By Friday I was in a deep depression. It was a wasted

27

exercise in self-pity; in the afternoon the telephone rang. Peter Edelman called from Washington to talk about my role in the campaign. It was wonderful news and I was manic again. I was wanted.

I would be designated director of state and local issues for the California primary campaign, responsible for developing Kennedy's stances on matters of vital interest to Californians, writing position papers, drafting speech materials, and — along with the press staff — manipulating and maximizing media coverage. That was the formal job description, but the Kennedy people had other, subtler, duties in mind as well, duties requiring a gift for disingenuousness.

The organization and operation of the California campaign were sensitive tasks. California was the prize that everyone expected would determine the nomination. Kennedy and McCarthy were likely to come into the June 7 primary with a mix of close victories and defeats in other states behind them. JFK's legacy of support in the largest state presumably made it Kennedy country, but California this year, along with most of the country, was volatile and unpredictable. It was essential to achieve a big win. With the momentum of that triumph, the campaign would confidently move into mop-up operations in the few remaining state primaries and conventions, and then on to the Chicago convention where Mayor Daley would deliver Illinois and, with the juggernaut now unstoppable, the nomination. But California was the key.

Apart from his own base of popular support in the state, Kennedy's biggest asset there was Assembly Speaker Jess Unruh, whom Kennedy had named chairman of his California campaign. Unruh had supported JFK and had publicly started drumming up support for another Kennedy presidency well before Robert had announced that he would run. But his bulky presence in the campaign was not an unmixed blessing, and the national campaign's senior staff people knew it. While they were grateful for Unruh's fidelity and admired his political skills, they also knew that he was a much-hated adversary of the California Democratic Party's ideological left wing, that he had his own large ambitions, and that he had a capacity for ruthlessness in pursuit of his ends that rivaled their own. Unruh was both a valued strongman and a potential bull let loose in Kennedy's political china shop; Kennedy's dilemma was how to exploit Unruh's power base yet keep him and his people from running amok and leaving ruin in his path. I was to have a role in solving that problem.

Standing short of six feet yet weighing about three hundred pounds, Unruh had come to be known as Big Daddy, a sobriquet that attested to his talent for gathering and wielding power as much as to his girth. Raising money from lobbyists and fat cats and storing it in a so-called Speaker's Fund that he invented but that subsequently became an institution, Unruh parceled it out at election time to his favored candidates. With his absolute control of immense amounts of cash, Unruh could make or break the career of virtually every aspirant to the Assembly in the state's Democratic districts. Those he favored with his largesse won; those he opposed lost. And once in office, the winners were forever beholden to Big Daddy, delivering their votes like automatons. When on rare occasions Unruh's enemies got elected, they found themselves assigned to obscure legislative committees, powerless and ridiculed until such time as they might repent, and, with promises of loyalty, receive his blessing.

Possessed of a dirty mouth whose flights of vulgarity cowed even the sleaziest of statehouse politicians, and driven by his own strange demons, Jess Unruh reigned as the unchallenged king and architect of the California legislature. Given the astuteness with which Unruh aggregated power, and the ruthlessness with which he exercised it, Richard Daley of Chicago, standing beside him, could be mistaken for a choirboy. Governor Pat Brown and his constituency of romantic, doctrinaire liberals hated Unruh; they hated him because he was obnoxious, but mostly they hated him because they didn't understand power and he did.

For all his crudities, Unruh was a genius. He made the California Assembly the most competent and responsible legislative body in the country and was himself one of America's greatest state legislators. He was an impassioned public servant who understood reality. If he unabashedly controlled people with his political money, and wielded his power with the bluntness of a club, he was also — as politicians go — scrupulously honest. Jess Unruh's political credo is best summed up by quoting his own deathless words when an interviewer asked him what the qualifications were for a good legislator in Sacramento: "If you can't accept the lobbyists' money, their liquor, and their women, and then vote against them, you don't belong up here." He was widely known as a man who followed his own pithy counsel.

Unruh wanted to be governor. With a Kennedy victory in California, achieved by a new statewide campaign organization chaired by Unruh and staffed by his people, the rotund speaker of the Assembly would be left equipped with an efficient and powerful machine in which to ride to his own triumph.

The Kennedys didn't care what Unruh would choose to do for himself in California with the spoils of a Kennedy victory — *after* the election. But they had to keep their California operation from looking as if it was being run by Big Daddy and his retinue of petty bosses. The romance and slogans, if not quite the reality, of the "New Politics" were abroad in America, and California was the center of the ferment. Political deals cut in smoke-filled rooms were supposedly out of fashion. In California particularly, where the rhetoric of reform was most shrill, the

Kennedy campaign had to have a New Politics sheen to it. Otherwise, the newly motivated idealistic young, as well as the liberal-left old pros of Alan Cranston's California Democratic Council, who had hated Unruh for years, would forgo the campaign, and the broad, inclusive base of support needed for a solid victory would be unattainable.

The plan was to let Jess Unruh and his troops screw together the assorted parts of the get-out-the-vote machine, raise money, and behind the scenes play political hardball with the state's old pros, while Kennedy and his people would build and polish the public façade — a shining crusade of social revolution and romance, led by a hero free of bossism and the old politics, and energized by the spirit of the people.

The Kennedys let Unruh name the managers of the northern and southern California campaign organizations and numerous supernumeraries throughout the state. They then moved deftly and swiftly to establish their own control of the important pressure points. Within a week of the opening of the California offices, old-line Kennedy men from across the country were in place. Claiming no titles, they announced that they were just there to "give a little help where needed" and, as old friends of Kennedy, provide a bit of coordination between the state and national campaign staffs. Armed only with their PT Boat 109 tie clasps from JFK's campaign, and a few casual references to the old days with Jack and/or Bobby, their authority lay in their vague membership in a mystique. By and large, they were political sophisticates who didn't depend on politics for a living, mostly volunteers on leave from law firms and businesses, who moved with the graceful authority of people who didn't need the jobs they presently held. Soon they were recognized everywhere as the de facto managers of the campaign, and Unruh's cadre of professional hangers-on weren't about to challenge them.

I was ideally positioned to maximize my role. With my Walinsky connection, I was viewed as a Kennedy loyalist, but I also was a Californian with an established relationship with some of Unruh's people. When Peter Edelman called to talk about my job in the campaign, he outlined a responsibility that was both exciting and sensitive. I was assigned to work with Ray King. King was an old-line Unruh operative who had been appointed northern California campaign manager. I had met him in 1966 when I had signed up to work for a year in the new War on Poverty. He had been deputy director of the Western Regional Office and I had been general counsel and special assistant for policy and plans. There had been millions of dollars to pass out to the new, volatile, largely black- and Chicano-run "community action" groups, and we had had a great deal of freedom to do what we wanted with the money. It was my first real taste of direct, personal power. King and I had vied for supremacy. Our styles had been different — he represented the heavy-handedness of the "Old Politics" and I fancied myself an elegant brigadier of the "New" — but we had stayed friends. Because of our old friendship he would welcome me, with the Kennedys' endorsement, in the senior policy job Edelman had outlined.

I would be perceived by King as one of his employees, an old and friendly colleague and therefore part of the Unruh apparatus; as such, I would be privy to thoughts and plans that might not be freely shared with Kennedy invaders from the East. In my official role, I would shape Kennedy's positions on issues to maximize his California appeal; in my unofficial role, I would be the national organization's agent within the Unruh apparatus, a bridge between the national and state campaigns — in short, a facilitator, an interpreter, and a spy.

I had a role that exceeded my wildest dreams. I was *the* Kennedy man in the California organization, a confidant of those closest to the prince, in a position to influence policy and wield power — all in a cause that, as I saw it, would renew America with justice, hope, and peace.

A couple of weeks into the campaign, a heavy roller in Kennedy's finance committee sought me out in the headquarters and invited me for a drink. He said he wanted to meet me because Chuck Spaulding, a senior Kennedy man from New York, had mentioned that Dick Smart was the only person on the California staff they knew they could trust. At the time, I hadn't even met Chuck Spaulding, and the incident confirmed my heady new status. Robert Kennedy was on his way and I was firmly on board.

Once Kennedy had made his decision, the pieces of the campaign were gathered from around the country and assembled with a speed and precision that could be achieved only by money, established political power, and an extraordinary level of emotional commitment by the Kennedy retinue's top echelon.

A few days after Edelman's first phone call, he called again and told me to fly to Los Angeles to meet with Kennedy's key people at the Ambassador Hotel. If there had been a meeting, it was over when I arrived at the appointed time. There was much milling around and animated conversation. Among those present were Steve Smith, Kennedy's brother-in-law and campaign manager, a man as crisply elegant as a freshly printed hundred-dollar bill; Chuck Spaulding, a diffidently patrician money man out of New York; Bob Fitzgerald, darkly handsome and aggressive, a young Kennedy cousin at the center of Boston's vaunted "Irish Mafia"; and half-a-dozen others.

I was introduced to somebody named John Seigenthaler, whose name had a vaguely familiar ring. Seigenthaler told me that he was going up to San Francisco to help out with the campaign and would appreciate it if I would join him on the flight to brief him on the situation there. I told him

I would be happy to, although not without a feeling of some resentment. I had evidently been summoned to Los Angeles not, as I had anticipated, to proffer my wisdom at a high-level strategy meeting, but to ride back on an airplane with some nondescript functionary.

John Seigenthaler was a curious animal among the company he was keeping. Craggy faced, with uninteresting and wrinkled clothes, wearing a haircut out of the fifties, and with the haggard look of a dust bowl refugee, he seemed light-years removed from the fashionable Boston–New York–Washington axis of the other Kennedy courtiers. His words came out not with a Kennedy urgency and crispness, but slowly and softly, a mixture of western twang and southern drawl that bespoke a schooling in Jim Nabors country. He was friendly, soft, and talked tired, an enigma who had no flash at all.

On the plane, all I learned was that he had come out from Tennessee for a while because "Bob" had asked him to lend a hand in California. That was hardly a biography, but Seigenthaler obviously thought the casual "Bob" a sufficient credential to seal an immediate rapport of political intimacy. He proceeded to run down a mental list of San Francisco political figures, asking my appraisal of each one. What was this one's motive for supporting Kennedy? What was that one's power base? Was he competent? Could so-and-so raise money, or contribute it himself? Who were his political allies? Could so-and-so be trusted?

What about Mo Bernstein? A dyed-in-the-wool Democrat with generally liberal sentiments, but a pragmatist rather than an ideologue, was my opinion. He paid lip service to noble political causes but real money to winners.

Ray King? The San Francisco campaign manager would do what Unruh told him to do, I thought. He'd work hard for the campaign, but his concern would be how he could parlay his manager's job into bigger things for himself in San Francisco politics.

John Warnecke? Warnecke, I said, struck me as largely uninterested in the substance of politics, and attracted less by the Kennedys' ideas than their cachet. He had partied with JFK, had been awarded some big government architectural commissions during the New Frontier, and was the family's choice to design the Kennedy Center in Washington. Whether out of idealism, or for fun and profit, he undoubtedly was a Kennedy loyalist and could be counted on to give some parties and raise some campaign money.

Adolph Schuman? With Mo Bernstein and Walter Shorenstein, he was a member of the troika of multimillionaires that controlled most of the heavy Jewish money that nourished San Francisco's Democratic politicians. A devoted Kennedy man, Schuman would do anything asked of him.

During the one-hour flight, the interrogation went on and on. Perhaps twelve or fifteen names were tossed at me for quick appraisal, with Seigenthaler now looking at me intently, now gazing out the window, as he listened to the answers, taking no notes, his only comments occasional, barely audible grunts. Some of the people I knew personally and others only by reputation, but in all cases I was confident that my answers had been incisive and accurate. Initially, I had been nervous at the drift of Seigenthaler's queries and constrained by an instinctive caution; but, as the relaxed voice had drawled on, I had, without realizing it, been massaged by its soft, subliminal authority and seduced into unguarded candor. The man was a total stranger; I didn't know what his own interests were, what he knew and didn't know, or what use he would make of what I'd told him. What I *did* know was that while I had lauded some of the subjects with unreserved praise, I had dissected quite a few more with some unkind cuts. My purpose had been honest helpfulness, not malice; nonetheless, passed on to the wrong ears, the blunt appraisals of some of the most powerful and egocentric people in San

35

Francisco could, if I were named as the source of them, finish me in the town.

And with that unsettling thought there came another. If this quiet, low-keyed man was in fact, as he so casually intimated, at the heart of the Kennedy apparatus, why had he had to ask me about longtime Kennedy intimates like Schuman and Warnecke? There was no reason why he should have known about many of the people on his list, but it was inconceivable that he didn't already know infinitely more about those two than I did. Was his interrogation really intended more as an appraisal of *me* than of its intended subjects? In quick retrospect, it seemed likely. Whatever my traveling companion's true motives, I knew that, in less than an hour, I had either established myself with him as a valued insider, or I had ruined myself by my indiscretions. As we approached the ground my stomach turned over, and it wasn't from air turbulence.

The old wave of anxiety, always so disproportionate to the relative pettiness of the problems that summoned it, was sweeping over me again. Firmly ensconced in an important political job, and blessed with my employer's glowing statements of confidence, I was assaulted, even before my first day of work, by the same old fear of a mistake or a misstep, of being misunderstood. My positive thoughts of the week just past, the thrill of the historic task that lay ahead, were now displaced by my recurring preoccupation — how to avoid the fatal error that I was always sure lurked around the next corner, waiting to devour both the image and substance of my life. For a few days I would again brood in one of the depressing valleys of that emotional roller coaster from which my psyche for years had been unable to escape. And while in that valley, my brain, as it always did during such dark periods, would focus not on the realities of duty, but on the creation of fantasized scenarios for my survival amidst myriad imagined threats and failures.

* * *

The following Monday morning, the core staff of the campaign met together for the first time in the newly opened headquarters, a huge, cold building on upper Market Street that had been an automobile dealership. The showroom, with its twenty-foot ceiling, had been partially partitioned into a dozen small cubicles for clerical workers and volunteers. A balcony, already divided into private offices, ran the length of the rear of the building. Soon the cavernous ground floor would be furnished with long portable tables full of typewriters, telephones, stacks of paper, and mimeograph machines. Crews of young volunteers would be folding mailers, stuffing envelopes, running off press releases, answering a dozen telephones that threatened to ring off their hooks, running about delivering messages, and generally dedicating themselves with awesome energy to the organized chaos of a big-time political campaign. Upstairs, removed from the bedlam, the "brains" would perform their more glamorous strategic functions — writing speeches; cutting deals with, and allocating money to, favored local pols; organizing fund-raising cocktail parties and dinners among the city's liberal-rich glitterati; cajoling the press for coverage; organizing get-out-the-vote efforts in the precincts; pasting together special interest committees of women, lawyers, minorities, labor leaders, environmentalists, and professors; in short, putting together the battle plans, money, and armaments that would make for a resounding victory.

We met in a large conference room at the end of the balcony. Josiah Beeman, a bald, three-hundred-pound Buddha who had left the Presbyterian ministry for politics, was there, representing Phil Burton, the brash and abrasive young congressman and San Francisco campaign chairman who later would become the Democratic whip, second in power only to Tip O'Neill. Libby Gatov, treasurer of the United States under JFK, an elegant woman

37

in her fifties, had come in from Marin County with wisdom and patrician charm. Millionaire Adolph Schuman, burning with intensity and devoid of small talk, was there to speak of money. Diane Feinstein, an attractive, rich woman in her early thirties who was married to a neurosurgeon, was there to organize women for Kennedy and raise money, her first serious step along a political road that eventually would take her to City Hall as San Francisco's first woman mayor. A feisty young woman named Sally Quinn, who years later would become a prominent journalist and marry *Washington Post* editor Ben Bradlee, had come out from Washington to work on publicity. Tom Sorensen, a University of California vice-president and the brother of JFK's counsel and speechwriter, was also present at that meeting, as well as a young international banker and a newly rich stock market speculator, who would serve on the finance committee, a hotshot reporter on leave from the *Chronicle*, who would run the press operation, and half-a-dozen others. The campaign was under way.

Ray King presided at the head of the table, introduced the players to each other, described their jobs, and announced that the same group would convene to report their activities every Monday morning at ten. John Seigenthaler sat quietly off to one side, unobtrusive, presumably listening, and saying very little.

At the campaign's second meeting, John Seigenthaler was sitting at the head of the table and a sullen, silent Ray King sat off to the side. There had been no announcement of a palace coup, no public embarrassments of King; one morning, Seigenthaler simply was *there*, the soft-spoken captain of Kennedy's praetorian guard sitting in the chair graciously usurped from Unruh's local retainer, ruling with assumed authority and without apology or explanation. King was left with the courtesy of his title and the nourishment of his salary and little else; the campaign had become unmistakably Seigenthaler's — which is to say

Kennedy's — show. And quite a show it was. His first edict was that we would not meet Monday mornings at ten, but every morning of the week at eight.

He had gotten his suit pressed and, although he nearly always looked a little tired, he acted and spoke with an easy precision that seemed to flow endlessly from some bottomless reservoir of energy. His few days of personal orientation, in the feigned posture of laid-back listener just hanging around to see where he might help out, were over; he moved through the campaign organization and the city's media-money-political establishment with a sureness of purpose and deftness of touch that made him a star within a week. The odd Tennessee drawl was still there, but now it shaped words of humor, wisdom, and clear orders that, despite their soft tone, left no doubt that their authority was forged from hard steel. Seigenthaler was a tough, nononsense operator with a brain that worked like a combined bear trap and sponge, and his best public weapon was a velvet, disarming charm.

By this time I was fully aware that John Seigenthaler was something much more than the nondescript, vaguely unsettling man I had flown into the city with only a few days earlier. He was not just a longtime Kennedy supporter from the sticks, but Robert Kennedy's closest friend in all the world — his conscience, confidant, number-one troubleshooter, and alter ego. In the bloodiest days of the civil rights movement, when black churches were torched across the South and black leaders murdered with impunity, it was John Seigenthaler, his top aide at the Justice Department, to whom Bobby had turned for counsel and courage. It was Seigenthaler who had climbed on a bus in Montgomery, Alabama, to accompany the freedom riders into town, who had dismounted first to confront the mob and announce himself as the representative of the attorney general of the United States, and who immediately had been clubbed to the ground with ax handles.

After John F. Kennedy's assassination, it had been Seigenthaler who had stood by the dead President's younger brother in his darkest hours. Now Kennedy had turned to him again when he needed a trusted troubleshooter to forge order out of potential chaos in the key state in his run at the presidency.

After the passing of my fear that I had ruined myself at our first meeting, Seigenthaler and I had become friends. Apparently, I had told him just the sort of things he wanted to hear; he trusted me in all matters, we exchanged confidences throughout the campaign, and I was given my head to range far and wide in functions well beyond my original mandate. We drank together, strategized together, and he gave me a larger office. With Walinsky and Edelman as my patrons I had felt well-positioned; now, with Seigenthaler as a daily colleague, the future possibilities were staggering. Walinsky and Edelman would have much to say about the policies of the Kennedy restoration; but nobody, I was certain, would have more to say than John Seigenthaler in the selection of those people from the campaign who would be awarded the new administration's fattest plums. I had become a senior employee, confidant, and drinking buddy of the best friend of the next President of the United States.

To be, in 1968, a thirty-six-year-old idealist hungry for power and drawn by the glamour of radical chic, and to have landed a key job in Robert Kennedy's fight for the presidency, was to feel that God, approving of your appetite and tastes, had favored you with a role in a historic morality play; a drama that, as the date of the California primary election approached, was unfolding with the certitude of ordained destiny. Kennedy's rhetoric had taken on a messianic ring, and we, his militant disciples, were infected with both the zealotry and the hubris of a Chosen People. It really wasn't possible — and at the time I didn't try — to sort out how much of my passion was born of an emotional commitment to Kennedy's proclaimed New Jerusalem of compassion, justice, and peace, and how much of it came from my own hunger for power and glamour. That is a kind of self-dissection that few in politics ever consciously undertake, and those who do usually are losers. Belief in one's superior claim to power is the essence of getting it; and that is a special arrogance which is helped along immeasurably by an absolute conviction that one's personal ambitions are of a piece with the public welfare. All people who are driven by political ambition see their motives as bound up in the interests of "the people," but never more so than in the Kennedy campaign. And as for the glamour of it all, that went with the turf.

If the campaign's rhetoric was infused with the spirit of Sparta, large numbers of its courtiers were voluptuaries with Roman tastes. Drawn by the magnetic aura of another Kennedy, the glitterati flocked into town from the East and Beverly Hills. By day I was a political operative preoccupied with strategizing and speechwriting; by night I became a social lion engaged in chic recreation with an entourage of Beautiful People playing their walk-on roles with dash.

At Tadich's grill I indulged in small talk about life at the top with Tom and Joan Braden. After adventures in the CIA, he had become a wealthy San Diego newspaper publisher. His wife had a friendship with Nelson Rockefeller. With his rugged good looks and her beauty and effervescent charm, they seemed the quintessential social register–cum–politics couple destined for glory in the new Kennedy administration. Rafer Johnson came to town in a tuxedo, showing that good-looking black Olympic decathlon champions were for Bobby Kennedy. Lance Allworth, the San Diego Chargers' star property, spoke for the country's white wide receivers. When David Susskind — in those days omnipresent and irrepressible as a television producer and talk show host — came to campaign, I hosted a small dinner of the elite in a private room at Jack's. In the city's bawdier days the building had been a first-class whorehouse, but now it was the preferred eatery for business and political dealmaking, for pretense, pontification, and dissembling; a perfect setting for the entertainments of another ilk of whoring, and David loved it. For the campaign's small, intimate fund-raisers for the high rollers — contributors of five hundred dollars or more — we went up to the mansions of Pacific Heights, where we ate hot hors d'oeuvres and drank premium liquor served by silent blacks in starched white jackets while earnest intellectuals from the East spoke fervently of Kennedy's passion for social justice.

My favorite soiree featured Arthur Schlesinger, Jr., JFK's resident academic turned courtier, come out again from academia — bow tie nattily askew, cigar in one hand and Chivas Regal in the other — to condemn irrational foreign adventures and promise that Bobby would get us out of the quagmire of Vietnam. Well, he of all people should have known; hadn't he, after all, been sitting with Rusk and McNamara and Bundy at the right hand of the older presidential brother when he led us deeper into the quagmire in the first place? But a good historian turned politician is nothing if not versatile in analysis and selective in memory, and, talking to Arthur privately in a remote corner of the elegant salon, I was suffused with an assuring feeling of kinship with that small tight world of erudition, wisdom, and charm that surrounded my candidate and now me.

These were wonderful months of deeply felt purpose, intense work, and sustained euphoria, when, more than at any other time of my life, I felt my talents worthy of my ambitions, and my ambitions capable of fulfillment. The glamour was a delicious frosting, but the cake that nourished the work was made of moral commitment and hard-edged ambition.

The Sunday before the California primary, although there was little that could still be done to affect the vote, Seigenthaler asked a handful of the senior staff to come into headquarters. It was a quiet morning bright with sunshine. Market Street, brimming with traffic during the week, was nearly empty except for families on their way to church and a few derelicts sleeping off Saturday night's drunk in doorways with their empty bottles clutched to their chests. Around ten o'clock, Seigenthaler walked in with Kennedy. During the previous months I had seen Kennedy dozens of times on television and, from a distance, at rallies and fund-raisers. But this was the first time that I had been with him up close since Walinsky had introduced us nearly a year before. Always wiry in body, and with a chiseled face that was all angles and very little flesh, Kennedy looked even skinnier than usual, frail and very tired. The campaign had taken a heavy toll. He walked around among the half-dozen of us and softly thanked us for our work, not as Caesar but as a worn-out colleague. The impassioned, sometimes strident crusader whom his adoring legions had made a demigod, looked at us with bloodshot eyes, whispered his few hoarse words of comradeship, and, shoulders sagging with fatigue, left to get a plane for Los Angeles, where he would spend the remaining two days.

It was a strange, moving encounter that left my eyes wet. For months the campaign we had run had been a juggernaut, and we had thrived on the unrelieved action and noise of righteous war. Now, with our leader's Sunday visit to his camp, cavernous and empty but for a handful of loyalists, it struck us for the first time that the battle was over. He had come not with raised arms, driven by the roar of the adoring crowds that followed him everywhere, but as an exhausted mortal, quiet and alone. In sadness we knew that, whatever glories would follow Tuesday's report of victory, we would never again in all our lives recapture the special joys of that wonderful fight. Suddenly his fatigue became our own.

I had one remaining job to do. Seigenthaler had asked me to give him a memorandum outlining responsibilities that I might assume for the balance of the campaign. Although the California effort was concluded, and nobody doubted either the outcome or the virtually irresistible momentum that the victory would generate, much work still had to be done in other states to nail down the nomination. With my roots in Utah and family connections there, I suggested that I be appointed Kennedy's representative to the Rocky Mountain states, advising and coordinating the local organizations in the last six weeks of struggle for convention delegates. Seigenthaler liked the idea and said he would get back to me the day after the primary. It was clear that I was no longer seen as just a good Kennedy man in California, but was being taken into the inner circle of the national organization. And with that, and with Kennedy's defeat of Nixon in November, I would be on my way to Washington.

On the first Tuesday of the sixth month of 1968, I slept late, voted at noon, returned home for a few more hours of recuperative sleep, and in the evening went to California Hall for a raucous victory party. All of my colleagues from the campaign were there, joined by a thousand others who had tirelessly toiled for Kennedy in the streets, all revelers come to celebrate their leader's triumph, their own good work, and the dawning of a new America. Long tables were heavy with food, and booze and beer were consumed with an abandon known only to political workers hot on the scent of victory. Several large television sets announced the returns throughout the evening and kept us in touch with the celebration of our Los Angeles comrades-in-arms at the Ambassador Hotel. As reports came in from precinct after precinct around the state, our enthusiasm mounted to fever pitch.

Close to midnight Kennedy came down from his suite to make his victory speech and we all crowded around the television sets. A few minutes later there came from the sets the sound of a small explosion. A single voice was heard to shout something, then came screams and bedlam. A television reporter shouted that he had heard gunfire. A camera zoomed in on a group kneeling around a prostrate figure. Robert Kennedy lay unconscious, his head resting on a bloodsoaked towel, with a bullet in his brain. He died a day later, and with him went what little was left of the lingering innocence of my youth.

A day or two after Robert Kennedy died I got a telegram from his widow inviting me to his funeral at St. Patrick's Cathedral in New York. I didn't attend; it was cheaper and easier to drink at home, and it was unnecessary to shave.

A few months later, *Esquire* published an elaborate four-color chart of the seating arrangements at St. Patrick's, with the names of the invited mourners displayed to show, by their assigned places in the hierarchy of mourning, their rank in the Kennedy pecking order. Ted Kennedy gave his brother an eloquent eulogy; *Esquire,* tastelessly but tellingly, published a graphic obituary of a presumptive government and slain ambitions. My name was well enough placed among the favored to confirm the personal triumph that might have been, and to deepen my bitterness that it would never be. I had expected an insider's seat at a President's inauguration; what I got instead was my name published in a generational death notice. I felt personally betrayed by history and, in the assassination's embittered aftermath, it was impossible for me — as I'm sure it was impossible for many others who had tied their destinies to another's star — to know which I despaired of the most, Kennedy's tragic fate or my own murdered dreams.

* * *

Sirhan Sirhan's bullet killed more than Robert Kennedy; it killed the better side of a generation's passion. Our spirit of renewal and idealism had been wounded with the assassination of Martin Luther King, and it died with Kennedy. The substance of our revolution — the *purpose* that had enlisted our passions — vanished as quickly as it had come. We found ourselves chic rebels without a cause, left only with a permissive new life-style taken up as an adjunct of our revolution's trashing of the past.

Within an incredibly short time the circle had closed. The crusade, born in a mood of moral outrage and disillusion, initially had manifested itself in open rebellion against American institutions and values, had matured into a responsible political movement, and — at a "victory" party in Los Angeles' Ambassador Hotel — had died as suddenly as it had been born. And the disillusion at the end was, if anything, deeper than at the beginning. Outrage had been displaced by cynical resignation.

I don't know why a political movement that I thought had historic dimensions, and my passion for what it represented, simply expired with the killing of a leader. It may have been because, from the beginning, it had been excessively fertilized by the romance of the Kennedy personality cult and thus represented far less than met the eye. It may have been because, notwithstanding our moral fervor, the troops' commitment had been invested with too heavy a dose of personal ambitions to be realized under a second Kennedy presidency — ambitions for glamour, glory, and influence that collapsed with the fallen prince. Or it may have been that, with the assassination of Robert Kennedy — the last of the three men whom liberal America had come to regard as the prophets of a new age of justice and moral fulfillment — our communal spirit simply suffered one too many wounds, a final trauma that crippled the will for continued engagement.

Whatever the reason, the legions returned to their universities and law firms, stripped of their briefly renewed capacity for belief. The American renaissance was not to be. For the agitators of the New Left, the assassinations seemed to confirm the futility of peaceful change through the mainstream political system and reinforced their cynicism. For me and my radical chic friends, the killing brought immediate despair and long-term malaise. Nothing that was to follow the disillusioning years of Lyndon Johnson, whose war policies had betrayed us and whose personal style had been an affront to the elegance of Camelot — not the years of Richard Nixon, whose corruption seemed to confirm our perception that the American system was full of dry rot; and not the years of Jimmy Carter, whom we saw as a restoration of that empty American sanctimony without substance that we had rejected in the first place — would offer anything to dispel the darkness and restore our lost fervor. For both the angry rebels of the New Left and the radical chic, the moral crusade and its hundreds of thousands of intense personal commitments were over. But the party that the voluptuous young had invited us to was just beginning.

If the Kennedy killing brutally ended a romantic chapter of my life, it, and the campaign experiences that preceded it, provided the seeds for some new beginnings. One was the definitive beginning of the end of my first marriage. My infidelities had started in New York and increased during our three years in San Francisco. Had they been the only problem, we could have lived with them. The new credo of sexual freedom was being loudly preached by the country's sophisticates, and San Francisco was their most prominent pulpit. My past sins now seemed sanctioned by both modern philosophy and high fashion, and, with a minimum of static, we came to an unspoken acceptance of the possibility of playtimes in other people's beds. And, although our interests and private thoughts had traveled gradually diverging paths since virtually the day of our marriage, we had settled into an affectionate, comfortable, and civil, if not always communicative, marriage.

For nine years, Arlene had been outwardly accepting. The periods of brooding and occasional complaints had become more frequent but, by and large, she still had played the role of dutiful, if increasingly silent, wife. Weekends had been good family times, with congenial dinners, games, television, and walks with our children in the park; but I had unconsciously shut her out of my "real" life. As she had become more inner-directed, I had become more convinced that she would never be able to understand or appreciate, let alone help me conquer, the world of wealth, fame, and power to which I felt ceaselessly summoned. And the more I had ignored her as ill-equipped to share my dreams and ventures, the less inclined she had been to try. It was as though we were trapped in a viciously spinning, expanding circle with our lives thrown to opposite places on its outer rim.

The Kennedy campaign was the beginning of the end of tolerance and of our marriage. It had been three months of seven-day workweeks, with nights of drinking and partying with campaign friends, almost always without Arlene. But it was all going to be over on election day, and I had promised her that I would be home by midnight.

She had come late to the victory party, where she had found me immersed in revelry. After a few minutes she took me aside and said she had to get out of the place. She was on the verge of tears and told me that, amidst all the celebration, she felt not joy but blackness, and some terrible sense of doom. I was put off by her intrusion of despair, refused to leave, and put her in a taxi.

When I finally did get home, it was three A.M. and I was drunk, red-eyed, and despairing. Sirhan Sirhan's shot had sent me to the nearest bar with a few despondent

48

friends where, already drunk from hours of mistaken celebration, we had tossed down glass after glass of bourbon, wept, and cursed life.

Arlene was awake and furious. It was one of only half-a-dozen times during our fifteen years together that the placid façade cracked, that her brooding gave way to unconstrained rage. She yelled that I was a thoughtless bastard and demanded an explanation of my drunken tardiness. I told her how I had been devastated by the shooting and had been drinking to drown the pain. She hadn't known about the shooting and she was devastated too. Arlene had loved Robert Kennedy and was horrified that her awful premonition had come to pass. She was also outraged that, whatever my pain, I hadn't seen fit to indulge in it at home. But why should she expect any consideration from me? — she'd never had any before. I fought back, yelled that she was insensitive, and said that there were more important concerns than the hour of my homecoming.

The next morning the field of battle shifted. Arlene wanted to know what I planned to do now. I had abandoned my practice for my bullshit political career and now that was gone too. We didn't have enough money to see us past the end of the month. Suddenly I was without a job and just what did I plan to do about it?

They were reasonable questions, but I protected myself from the immediate harsh realities of our situation by enveloping myself within the cloud of tragedy. Without understanding or mercy, I verbally flogged her for her shallowness. A great man had been wounded, probably mortally, the whole country feared for his life and for its future, it had been only hours since I had been struck in the deepest guts of my soul, and here she was interrogating me about our financial security. Had she no sensitivity?

Not for that line, she didn't; not with all that had gone before. In my frenetic search for the quickest path to power, I had taken five jobs in the years since law school, and had not consulted her about any of the moves until after I had already made the decisions in my own mind. Each exciting new opportunity had been announced with great flair as a critical step up the ladder that eventually would take us together to the stars, and — to all outward appearances — she had trusted my motives and judgments despite her hurt at being excluded from the thoughts that made them. Now there was no attempt even at the appearance of trust. To Arlene (and now to me, although I could never admit it to her), it looked as though, with each foot of ascent up the ladder, some enemy — which now seemed to be Fate itself — had been cutting a foot off the bottom, leaving me in a state of constant climbing while getting nowhere.

Arlene had had it with her role of bit player in my ongoing drama of cosmic dreams and miscarried ambitions. More than anything else, she wanted to know who *she* was, to be able to define herself by some identity beyond just that of somebody's wife. It was an urge that had been building for a long time. The Kennedy campaign was merely the catalyst that accelerated the ferment.

Arlene had returned to college in San Francisco to get the degree she had had to give up when I was in law school and she was pregnant with our first child. At San Francisco State, she had distinguished herself, confirming her suspicions that she was much smarter than I had encouraged her to believe, just at the time when Friedan, Steinem, Greer, and Millet were raising the consciousness of America's women, eloquently teaching the truth that they no longer had to live in a male-imposed state of economic, intellectual, and emotional servitude. I had actually been delighted, hoping that, in her newly discovered confidence, there was a basis for the partnership in adventure I had told myself I always wanted with a woman. But if that had ever been possible, it was too late. There had been too much past to deal with — too many indignities that I had imposed upon her, too many scars, and too many habits for me to unlearn.

Arlene and I would live together seven more years with reasonable affection and mutual love for our children, but with the wall that divided our understanding growing ever higher. For a time, I settled into making money and building security. I bought her the house she wanted; it comfortably sheltered our bodies but not her awakened spirit.

The Kennedy campaign not only brought the tacit truth of my long-deteriorating marriage into a state of open acknowledgment, it also propelled me into unreserved pursuit of sensual and material delights. My appetites had been well served by the campaign, the chic recreations that once had been occasional indulgences had become an addiction, and I wasn't about to kick the habit of living well. An assassination had robbed me of my immediate political career but had left me with my tastes, a new sense that I belonged in the world that indulged them, and, paradoxically, a ticket to pay for them.

Arlene need not have worried about where the next job would come from, for Mel, the international investment banker who had sought me out when he learned of my closeness to the Kennedy insiders, was there to pick up the pieces of my ruin. The Kennedy campaign had bequeathed me two new friends who would affect the rest of my life. They shared my tastes for haute cuisine, fine wines, celebrity, and the company of the powerful — and they had the money for it. For the next fifteen years, Mel, Michael — in the process of making a fortune on the stock market — and I would be an inseparable trio of bon vivants, bound together by the emotional roots of our friendship in the campaign and by our common lust for the sweet life, traveling at breakneck speed through the city's fashionable restaurants, its women, and its drugs.

Michael, at forty, was fast becoming one of the hottest

items among the city's nouveau riche, and was doing it not only with money but with class. Dashing, rich, and gifted with a seductive charm that seldom varied regardless of the audience, he provided salutary counterpoint to Mel's occasional lapses into vulgarity after too much scotch; in Michael's company, Mel felt closer to arrival at his place among the wealthy and civilized, an almost-social lion justified in his taste for expensive wines.

Mel was not quite rich yet, but he was getting there. He solidly controlled the thriving young investment banking company he had founded, and blessed himself with an unlimited expense account. Theoretically accountable to a board of directors, he had stacked it with a sufficient number of docile types to ensure that, with his persuasive talents, he could justify virtually any expenditure and seldom cause a rumble. A week after Kennedy was killed, Mel retained me, as a full-time consultant to his company in Palo Alto, paying me as much as anybody there except himself. I was to be responsible for marketing and long-range planning.

I was hardly an investment banking expert; I knew nothing about the business and cared less, but to Mel that was a virtue. He saw the company as his short-term means to a larger end, and persuaded himself that a young renaissance man of large vision, who conveniently shared his tastes, could help him get there. With our combined imagination, daring, and hard work, we would expand the company, sell it, cash out with fortunes, and go on to greater, albeit undefined, adventures.

It was a nicely romantic idea, but quite without substance. Mel was on an ego trip, I needed a job, and we relished each other's company.

Mel was a collector of people. His desire for money and power matched my own, and — unlike mine — it was accompanied by the temperament and talent for getting them. But with all of that, he had a darker, fearful side that manifested itself through a sharp division of his world into friends and enemies — with no room for ambiguities in between. He loved and hated with a passion, and San Francisco's business and social circles reciprocated; you either loved Mel or you hated him. Seeing a world full of "assholes" (his invariable expression of contempt) and feeling beleaguered by enemies and fools, he surrounded himself with a small circle of loyalists chosen for their present status or promising futures, hip images that by association would reflect well on his own, hedonistic tastes, and with a talent for sustaining an apparently uncritical love of Mel.

It was an oddly eclectic group. A couple of frequently stoned congressmen; a rock musician en route to stardom and drug addiction; an already addicted interior designer; a sturdy young carpenter with a taste for cocaine; a fashionable drug dealer; a rock concert management functionary who got Mel premiere tickets to prestige events and introduced him to groupies; a handsome young heir to a vast fortune and his stunningly beautiful wife, who jogged a lot and spent much of the rest of their time sharing with Mel the wisdom of Jung and the mysteries of the collective unconscious.

I was the new discovery — the bright young dilettante and political dabbler elevated to the position of philosopher/provocateur and house wit.

One night during the peak of the campaign's euphoria, Mel and his new girlfriend had introduced me to Sergeant Pepper's, the city's hottest new discotheque, where the young gathered in undulating celebration of the Beatles. It had quickly become a hangout for the three of us, and now it became the place where we danced, drank, and smoked our way back to vivacity.

The marijuana helped. I had had my first toke of marijuana the year before when it was introduced to me by a couple of black activists in Los Angeles with whom I was negotiating a multimillion-dollar federal antipoverty grant. In the ensuing months I had shared two or three joints offered surreptitiously and with great drama by hip adventurers living on the cutting edge of San Francisco's fresh new era of drugs, sex, and "raised consciousness." I had enjoyed my few early adventures with the gentle herb, but had never considered making it an integral part of my life-style. In the company of Mel and Nina, however, the pot did wondrous things for me. Mixed with Jack Daniels, it soothed the pain in my psyche, and my anxieties were dispelled with an easy, careless laughter that came even when nothing much was really funny.

The disco became transformed into a world of magic. The new music's sensual beat boomed from loudspeakers to ear to brain, where, enriched by pot's chemistry, they were transmitted to groin with a wonderful sexual clarity. Overhead, a huge ball with a façade of multifaceted cut glass slowly revolved while half-a-dozen spotlights, their hues programmed to change with the beat and volume of the music, bathed the undulating bodies below in waves of shifting color that caressed them into even deeper union with the mesmeric rhythms of guitar and drum. But when the rock beat hardened and the strobe came on to fill the room with pulsating flashes of hot white light, the sensual provocations that had preceded it seemed like foreplay. Under the light's rapid-fire bursts, women's faces became all flickering shadows playing on bleached ivory surfaces, with mascaraed eyes turned hollow and red lips turned black around gleaming wet teeth, ghostly apparitions of bloodless loveliness beckoning one to the delights of electric sex unburdened by the complexities of thought and soul.

The pot made even brighter the darts of light that danced off the girls' spangled tank tops. Their braless breasts were bouncier, their jeans tighter, the cheeks within more firmly rounded. Dancing through the night I felt as though I had electric shoes. One night early in July, I took a nineteen-year-old with black hair down to her waist home to her water bed in a one-room flat in the Haight-Ashbury. We smoked a joint, drank some Gallo's burgundy, and under a huge poster of Mick Jagger, and with every cell alive to youth's precocious touch, I first savored the delights of pot-spiced sex.

At a time in my life when heavy thought came much too often, marijuana bestowed the blissful gift of mindlessness, sending the senses soaring while it numbed the brain. Under its spell the world looked at once a safer and more luscious place. For Mel and me, it became an access ticket to the exotic new world being shaped by the unabashed and hedonistic young. In 1968, Mel was forty and I was thirty-six, members of a transitional generation in limbo between our own parents' traditional values and the new ethos of guiltless self-indulgence. What was happening among the young looked to us like high adventure for both the body and the spirit. With newly bitter memories of our own repressed youth, we damned the unfairness of our having been born fifteen years too soon.

With pot in our brains we deciphered the Beatles' cryptic messages with the acuity of twenty-year-olds — as though the years of board meetings, mortgages, and dental bills had never intervened to mar the clarity of innocent understanding. We became as young and hip as anybody. And, with our eyes glassy, beatific smiles frozen on our faces, and a few extra joints in our pockets to share with soul mates, the authentic young accepted us; if we weren't exactly one of their own, we were certainly turned-on senior citizens who were a gas to boogie with — especially when Mel plied them with pot and paid for their drinks.

Mel's girlfriend Nina was an excellent guide for our trip into youth's brave new world. The daughter of a wealthy Park Avenue dentist, she was one of thousands of young people who, suddenly resentful of their comfortable lives,

55

migrated en masse to San Francisco and its promises of liberation. When her marriage fell apart, she'd gone west with her twin boys. Mel had found her serving cocktails at a hip East Bay rock spot.

With Nina, every event in life was described in the argot of a new clarity — an "upper" or "downer," "right on" or "far out." Being quick learners, Mel and I soon could tell which was which, and we even learned what was and was not a "turn on." When the business day was done, she promptly got Mel out of pinstripes and into factory-faded designer jeans, silk shirt open to the navel, and gold chains, and off we would go into the rocking night. We were always ready to travel fast, but in Nina's company the pace was even faster. Mel had had two heart attacks before he was thirty-five. Nonetheless, he felt compelled to keep moving with the hot woman sixteen years his junior. If Nina could smoke one pack, he could smoke two; if she could handle four scotches, he could handle six; if she could dance through an entire night, he could dance forever — or however long it took to keep her from gyrating with one of the lank, finely muscled blacks wearing outrageous silks, white shoes, and rakish fedoras, whom she loved to entice onto the dance floor to keep Mel nervous. I had a healthy heart and my weight was down, but it was a challenge to keep up with the two of them.

In mid-July, Ted Sorensen's brother, Tom, telephoned me at the office. Tom and I had become close friends during the Kennedy campaign. He said that Alan Cranston, who had won the Democratic nomination for U.S. senator in the June primary, needed a speechwriter, and wanted to know if I would like the job.

I was hesitant to take it. Cranston, who had served as state controller, was a founder and leader of the California Democratic Council, a group of liberal ideologues whose influence had peaked with Pat Brown's election as governor. But Ronald Reagan had subsequently beaten Brown, and it appeared that the state was on a general drift to the right. Cranston seemed problematical himself. He had previously taken a shot at the other senatorial seat, but had lost it when the Kennedy forces sent former JFK press secretary Pierre Salinger carpetbagging into the state to snatch it away. And now he seemed set up to lose the next general election to his right-wing challenger, state school superintendent Max Rafferty.

In the pantheon of American demagoguery, Max Rafferty in his short career as California's superintendent of education was already on his way to earning an elevated place alongside Huey Long, Father Coughlin, and Joe McCarthy. A riveting orator given to flights of inflammatory rhetoric, he had used his "educator's" platform to attribute every ill in American society, from low student performance to high crime rates to antiwar protests, to Communists and their liberal sympathizers. He had the political support of the more moderate Reagan, and the financial support of the southern California fat cats — Henry Salvatori, Justin Dart, Holmes Tuttles, and a handful of other multimillionaires who had become the preeminent bankrollers of the California Republican Party's newly robust right wing.

If Rafferty was an unconscionable demagogue, Cranston at least had the virtue of never having raised an audience's temperature by *any* means, fair *or* foul. He had a reputation as a hardworking, decent, single-mindedly political man, who, for all his considerable acumen and worthy convictions, was an incurably boring speaker. Although often provocative in content, his speeches were delivered with a flatness and disregard for emotional inflection that made them a guaranteed cure for insomnia.

Bland and colorless, Cranston as a Senate candidate didn't even generate any real enthusiasm within his own party except among a few old loyalists and liberal ideologues. He'd have trouble raising money; and, even if he could get enough to finance a decent campaign, what would the campaign have to sell to the starstruck, celebrity-conscious California electorate that had given the country tap dancer George Murphy and now Ronald Reagan? Rafferty was already a media star of sorts; on television he would come across as sizzling beefsteak; by comparison Alan Cranston would look like refrigerated pablum. So ran the conventional wisdom.

At that particular time I was reluctant to make another job change to go into a campaign that was doomed to disaster. It had started to sink into my mind that, for whatever reason, I had begun to pile up a record of mis-carried adventures, near misses of the big success target. I liked what Cranston stood for, but that was hardly the issue; I didn't need to be associated, either in my mind or in reality, with another loss, not even another one that would be somebody else's fault.

But there were some offsetting considerations to think about. For one, there was the problem of my consulting job with Mel's company. However voluptuous my nights, I spent half my days trying to figure out something useful to do, and the other half doing marginally useful things in which I had no interest at all. I sorely missed the en-ergizing pace and excitement of politics. Despite the Kennedy campaign's bitter end, I had been bitten by the bug and thoroughly infected with the political virus. There was the very remote possibility, I thought, that, despite the unhappy early polls and the political seers' uniform prophecies of Cranston's impending doom, the man might pull a rabbit out of his hat and win. Or Rafferty, in his wildness, might commit a fatal faux pas. Politics was full of accidents and stupidities that converted sure winners into losers, and miraculously raised the politically dead and made them victors. The odds were extraordinarily long, but if Cranston somehow were to pull it off, it wouldn't be bad to be aboard.

Beyond the calculations of self-interest was the fact that, with or without a candidate to attach myself to, I had become emotionally enlisted in the battle to defend the ramparts of liberal humanism against revived hordes of selfish conservatives and Philistines. Out of the ashes of what had been thought a political funeral pyre, the specter of Richard Nixon was again rising to claim, of all things, the presidency that, with Kennedy's assassination, looked more and more like a Republican prize. California had become a battleground of the country's philosophic and moral extremes. As much as we, in our liberal orthodoxy, had ridiculed George Murphy and his Hollywood friend Reagan, as much as we had throughout his career hated Nixon, Max Rafferty, more than any of them, symbolized the growing menace of the far right. Even with a boring candidate, the Cranston battle promised to be exciting, a watershed of California's political future, and maybe the country's.

I decided to talk to Mel about the offer. His reaction was quick and predictable — "It's a hell of an opportunity; I think you should take it." Mel looked for opportunities to extend his political tentacles wherever he could find them. If, as my patron, he let it be known that he had given me a leave of absence to help Cranston out, and by some fluke Cranston won, it would be a score for Mel. "And Richard, if Cranston *does* win, it'll be a damn good thing for you, whatever you decide to do after that. Cranston ain't Kennedy and the Senate ain't the presidency, but having a U.S. senator owing you can't hurt." Mel's sophistications always seemed to be directly to the point.

There remained the question of financial security. Although Arlene had disliked Mel from the start, she had heaved a great sigh of relief when I went to work for his

59

company. International investment banking had an aura of respectability and stability about it, and by now she didn't much care what I did so long as it brought in predictable money and appeared to end a life of professional nomadism. Now I had to go through the unpleasantness of announcing a job change all over again, while convincing her that I wasn't putting the family in financial jeopardy. Mel said not to worry about it. When the campaign was over I could return to his company and, after a couple of more months for the staff to get used to me, he would change the "consultancy" to a senior vice-presidency, and I would be a full-fledged, eminently secure investment banker.

Arlene greeted the announcement with disgust but resignation. The consultant fees I would get from the campaign were substantial and the Mel connection would, if need be, guarantee the future. She registered a pro forma protest when I told her that, except for weekends, I would be living in Los Angeles for three months. Her passionless reaction brought both a sense of relief and a twinge of sadness. If I felt a moment of regret it quickly passed. I packed my bags, kissed Arlene and the children good-bye, and flew to Los Angeles.

The campaign headquarters was on Wilshire Boulevard, a short walk from the Ambassador Hotel, where Kennedy had been shot, and not far from the glitter of Beverly Hills.

I went there directly from the airport and introduced myself to Tom Moore, the campaign manager, and Lu Haas, the press secretary, both seasoned war horses from Pat Brown's halcyon days, now working together again in what looked to be California liberalism's last hurrah. Surprisingly, the mood of the place was very upbeat. I attributed the optimism to politicians' incurable penchant for always foreseeing their man's victory, however bleak the objective outlook. But even if the good cheer rested on a foundation of quicksand, I got caught up in it and was anxious to go to work.

Moore introduced me to Allyn Kreps, an old family friend of Cranston's who had been appointed campaign chairman with plenary authority over every aspect of the operation. He was in his early thirties and had become a partner in one of Los Angeles' two biggest corporate law firms at an indecently early age. Kreps looked and acted like a storm trooper colonel, utterly in command without subtlety, tact, or humor. It was instantly obvious that Moore and Haas disliked Kreps intensely and that he returned the feeling.

He took me into his office alone and immediately made it known that he wasn't happy to see me. He didn't know anything about me, I had been thrust into the campaign by some of Cranston's northern California friends, and, anyway, he didn't think the campaign needed a full-time speechwriter; he had a stable of bright young writers back at his law firm who could crank out speeches. But I was there, and he supposed he would give me a tryout.

A few months earlier that kind of greeting would have plunged me into anxiety and I would have muttered that I was grateful for the chance. But my success in the Kennedy campaign, and the fact that I had been ambivalent about the job in the first place, emboldened me to strike back. "Mr. Kreps," I said, "I really don't know who you are either, but I was told I was coming down here on Alan Cranston's authority to write his speeches. I happen to be the best political speechwriter in the state, and I also happen to be a very busy man who doesn't need this job. And I certainly am not down here for a tryout. So I think the best thing for me to do is walk out of here right now and get a plane back to San Francisco."

To my amazement, the storm trooper folded. "Well, you don't need to be hasty," he said. "This isn't exactly the way I had planned to staff the organization, but you do come highly recommended and I'm sure it'll work out. The one thing that is important, though, is that you understand who is running this campaign. I'm the person — the *only* person — who sets policy."

"I'll be glad to cooperate with you," I said. "But as far as my job is concerned, Alan Cranston is running the campaign. I intend to plan the speeches with him directly, and I expect to write them without interference."

"Well," Kreps responded, "it's not going to be that clearcut, but I'm sure we'll work well together."

That was a statement that to me signaled a modest victory and I was proud of my performance. I felt that the insecurities that had so often plagued me in similar situations had been subdued once and for all. Now all I had to do was ensure that my performance matched my posture. Kreps took me into Cranston's office and left us alone for half an hour.

Alan Cranston in person matched his media image — bland. But he was even more off-putting in a private one-on-one encounter. There was a hint of warmth in the eyes, but everything else was cold as ice. His welcome and his statement that he was glad to have me aboard obviously were genuine, but lacking in the heartiness that I had become accustomed to in politicians. He spoke in mumbled monosyllables, his speech unadorned by wit or even a pro forma pass at feigned camaraderie.

We talked for a while about the strategies of the campaign and the kinds of speeches he wanted — all of them framed within the general themes of peace and social justice. I had to get to work immediately. The Democratic state convention in Sacramento was just over a week away, and Cranston was scheduled as the principal speaker. He thought that maybe he would like to give a speech on Vietnam, but he wasn't quite sure. It wasn't clear which way the middle class was leaning on the issue — particularly in California, where antiwar sentiment was being vented most visibly by scruffy, drug-loving hippies and long-haired students who were reviling their parents' values.

His natural instinct was to take a strong moral position against the war. This was opposed by Kreps, who had cautioned that the risks of such a position were too great, particularly with an opponent like Rafferty.

"Well," Cranston finally said, "let's take a crack at a draft of a Vietnam speech and see what it looks like."

"How strong do you want it?" I asked.

"Oh, strong," he said. . . . "Well, not *too* strong."

I sought out Haas, asked for a desk and a typewriter, and went to work. We were at a point of daily escalation of the war with no visible return; and we were supporting what seemed to me, and many Democrats, corrupt regimes. The speech, a long one, was finished the following afternoon. It was an attempt to analyze the course of events and remind America of its idealism. It began "The Vietnam war is a moral outrage" and continued in that vein with a sharp attack on President Johnson's policy and our failure to abide by the Geneva accord's provision for nationwide elections in a unified country. American soldiers should be brought home. I put one copy of the draft on Kreps's desk and the other on Cranston's.

The following morning, Kreps stormed into my office in a rage, demanding to know just what the hell I thought I was doing. "This speech is crap," he said. "Do you know what Rafferty will do with this? He'll crucify us. We've got enough of a problem with Cranston's reputation as a softheaded liberal without *this*. It makes him look like a Communist dupe and Rafferty'll tear him apart. Rewrite it. And rewrite it *responsibly*."

"I'll rewrite it after I have Cranston's reaction," I said.

"You mean to tell me that Cranston has a copy of this?"

"Of course; he is the one who gives the speeches, isn't he?"

"Goddammit, I told you that all speech drafts are to go through me."

"And so they will, but copies will also go to the candidate at the same time; that's a more efficient process, don't you think?" I had made my point regarding protocol and hence, indirectly but clearly, had staked out my claim for a particular power niche in the campaign. Now, I thought it prudent to try to pierce the totalitarian façade and win some respect, if not affection, with a little reason.

"Allyn, if you've got a little time, sit down and let's talk about this. You are running the campaign, and I accept that. At the same time, Cranston is entitled to a variety of views, and if you're going to have the best possible campaign, you shouldn't try to cut him off from them. As for the speech itself, Cranston isn't going to win by coming across as a moderate on *any* issue. You're going to win by polarizing this campaign on *all* issues, not just the war, but social and economic issues as well. Given Rafferty's nature, let's *make* Cranston a target by letting him say what he really believes — I don't think you're going to be able to stop him from doing that anyway. Besides, this speech happens to be the truth, and even in politics that might not hurt."

Kreps sat quietly for a minute, then finally said, "Well, in general, you may have a point, but not where Vietnam is concerned. The issue is too volatile, and I'm not going to let Cranston get out on a limb. The speech isn't badly written, but it's too flamboyant and too risky. You'd better get to rewriting it, because Cranston's not going to give it or anything like it."

Haas, Moore, and I accompanied Cranston to the Sacramento convention. He delivered the attack on America's Vietnam policy virtually word for word. The Cranston-Rafferty battle was the only interesting political game going on in the state, the news media had descended on Sacramento in droves, and the speech, coming from quiet, cautious Alan Cranston, electrified an otherwise dull convention and set the stage for a vitriolic campaign.

That night Lu Haas brought Tom Brokaw, a pleasant, good-looking newsman in his late twenties, into my Sacramento motel room. He was a political reporter for a Los Angeles television station who wanted a background briefing on the campaign, and particularly on the Vietnam speech. We chatted for half an hour about Cranston's Vietnam position and other campaign issues, and initiated a relationship that, over the years, would ripen into friendship. A little over a decade later, he would be national anchorman on NBC's "Nightly News."

Nobody suggested that Cranston had suddenly caught charisma, but he was widely praised for his courage. And barely a week later, Rafferty, as we had hoped, responded with outrageous excess, accusing Cranston of nothing less than treason.

Taking the bait, Rafferty plunged headlong into the trap of his own undisciplined mouth, and I quickly cranked out a rejoinder — a Cranston news release in which he thanked his opponent for putting him in the august company of Republican Senators Hatfield and Percy, who had taken similar positions, as a "member of Max Rafferty's club of Distinguished American Traitors." The press had a field day with the exchange, with all but the most right-wing papers scorching Rafferty for his demagoguery.

The early opinion polls had shown Rafferty to have a substantial lead, but, with only one bell-ringing speech and Rafferty's stumble, Cranston already had begun to turn a bad situation around. The next California poll showed the gap closing. I wouldn't get another hard word from Kreps and, after a time, we even became friends.

Money had been tough to raise but, with Cranston's fortunes suddenly brightened, the fair-weather liberal millionaires of Beverly Hills, Malibu, and Bel-Air were finally able to locate their checkbooks, and the cash started rolling in. When the smart money started placing Cranston bets, for the first time I really dared to believe that my growing hope for a win might be more than a pipe dream.

As our campaign was getting richer, Rafferty's was getting poorer. On issue after issue, in speech after speech, he continued to indulge his penchant for rhetorical excess, making Cranston's blandness look positively like high statesmanship. There were signs that Reagan was getting nervous and, as graciously as possible, was trying to put some distance between himself and his candidate. Soon, a couple of fat cats resigned from Rafferty's finance committee. They wanted a right-wing senator, but one with some class. Rafferty was becoming an embarrassment.

With a real prospect of victory, the campaign became great fun. Cranston began inserting terribly bad jokes in his prepared texts, eliciting from his audiences good-hearted groans more often than laughs, but nobody minded; we were on a roll. Glossy fund-raising parties proliferated in Beverly Hills, and again I was mixing with the rich and the glamorous, only more so. If the cream of San Francisco society thought they were rich, they didn't know what rich was. Beverly Hills money had a brighter sheen and there was tons more of it.

There was a stunning, black-tie fund-raiser at the Century Plaza, and Melina Mercouri, making her rounds as a crusader against Greek fascists, was my dinner partner. At the campaign office, I found Linda, a beautiful blond volunteer with a robust sexual appetite, an elegant Beverly Hills pad, and an endless supply of fine pot. She knew all the best restaurants and the glitterati who frequented them. By September the campaign and its perquisites had become a ball. Again full of what seemed like infinite energy, I was living life to the hilt. Days of nonstop work; evenings of parties and dining in restaurants whose prices guaranteed their exclusivity, always followed by nights of pot-enhanced lovemaking in Linda's bed; Sunday afternoons sitting with Kreps, Haas, and Cranston on the sun-bathed deck of the presumptive new senator's Bel-Air house, planning the week's strategy and relishing my unambiguous position as valued counselor to the mighty. The power rush had returned and I savored it as I did the rarest of wines. If, in my sanguine mood, I mistook consumption of power's trappings for possession of its reality, that was a distinction I wasn't interested in clarifying; it was enough just to enjoy the fine feeling.

In early September Michael telephoned me from San Francisco. A couple of years earlier, a lawyer friend of his had taken up car racing, and he was driving the next weekend at Laguna Seca — the big time. Michael wanted to know if I could break away from the campaign for a couple of days to attend the race. I could and I would. The track was just a few minutes from Carmel, the artsy paradise on the Pacific; the weekend would give me a reunion with Michael and Mel, and a couple of days with Arlene.

As the campaign had progressed, I had started to forgo even the weekend flights home; the delights of Beverly Hills were not easily interrupted by the call of domestic duty. Either I had begun to miss Arlene or I was feeling guilty; I wasn't sure which. The Carmel weekend would give us a little idyllic time together. Despite my blissful immersion in Beverly Hills pleasures and the renewed thrill of politics, and despite the slow withering of our marriage, there remained a vestige of caring. Of late, during the few nights when I had been in my hotel room sipping bourbon alone instead of smoking pot in Linda's bed, old memories had pierced through the pink haze of my glamorous new life, evoking sentiments of simpler times when love had seemed possible and my marriage had looked to be the path for finding it. A sunny afternoon in June, with final exams over, parking by a stream in the

67

Utah mountains in a 1946 black Dodge sedan and, with caresses and young kisses, arousing a sheltered, pretty eighteen-year-old brunette to her first true passion. Our marriage a year later, during a Christmas break at Yale, with my gentle father guiding us through our vows. Our first child, Ursula, playing on the floor of one of the tin-roofed Quonset huts that housed married students in those days, her tiny body warmed through the vicious New Haven winters by the heat of a coal-burning stove, while Arlene, in uncomplaining servitude to a student budget, concocted the stews and spaghetti sauces that would see the family through to richer times. The early New York days, before the beginning of disillusion, when all good things still seemed possible between us and we decided to have another child. Lisa's arrival, with her mother's brown hair and dark eyes in perfect counterpoint to Ursula's blondness, a wiry, tightly wound bundle of energy to balance her sister's soft poetry. There had been long hikes in the mountains with our children and picnics and camping trips, and some nice dinners out with just the two of us. Yes, even in the years of disintegration there had been many good times. And, if the passion had slipped away, there had been love and affection, and the sex had been good. If only she hadn't insisted on wearing that chintzy sequined black-taffeta dress to the law firm's Christmas ball at the Colony Club, I had often thought as I mourned the promising New York years that had slipped away, unfulfilled. I had warned her that a leftover rag from her junior prom wasn't going to make it among the silks and satins of my colleagues' wives. This wasn't a dance in a Utah college gymnasium; it was Park Avenue, for God's sake. But, with her unfailing eye for the budget, she had saved a few dollars; I had felt humiliated and feared that she would never understand what it took to make it in the world I had chosen. Yes, that dress was what really started us rolling downhill; if it hadn't been for that goddamn dress, things might have gone differently.

Although I had come to know better in the succeeding years, I couldn't erase the memory of that unreasonable feeling of embarrassment. Arlene had been perfectly happy in an old dress if it meant we could pay the next month's bills. Even then, barely out of law school, I had started spending money we didn't have on the theory that an affluent social façade was at least as critical to professional success as inner substance.

After all these years I wasn't about to retreat from luxury to simplicity, but maybe she could see that it was possible for her to share and enjoy the bounties of my full new life. Maybe — if I really *tried* — we could recapture some of the long-lost romance and make a go of it. The race weekend was worth a shot. We could spend a couple of hours at the race, have a dinner with Michael and Mel, and spend the rest of the time alone together, retrieving the good memories, ignoring the bad ones, and maybe dredging up a hope for the future. The bourbon had oiled my sentimentality, and the scenario seemed plausible.

It was a nice idea, but it didn't quite work out. From Friday night through Monday morning, our merry group sustained an orgy of food, liquor, marijuana, and high fun in the classiest restaurants and watering holes in Monterey and Carmel, interrupted only by brief snatches of sleep and a few hours at the track. Mercifully, in the first fifty yards of the race, Michael's friend's Porsche broke its transmission, freeing up the rest of the day for continued revelry. I quickly forgot the planned walks with Arlene on Carmel's snowlike sands, the intended quiet times when we would rekindle our expired love. Our trips to bed, anticipated as times of sexual bliss away from the children, became instead brief periods of recuperation for the next rush of group recreation. I had a wonderful time; it seemed that wherever I spent my days now — whether in San Francisco, Los Angeles, or a quaint ocean village — the sweet life abounded. Arlene drank and laughed with us and seemed to get along with Michael and Mel and their women. I was pleased that she apparently had come to share my appetite for life's finer times.

As it happened, she was not amused. I drove her back to San Francisco, where, in a voice dripping with acid, she thanked me for our *wonderful* weekend. I asked her if she wasn't going to drive me to the airport for my flight back to Los Angeles. She told me to take a cab. "I'm sure you can afford it," she said.

Some seven weeks later Alan Cranston was elected U.S. senator from California and again I felt myself a hero. The morning after the election, Cranston flew to San Francisco for a press conference, then took me to lunch at Trader Vic's with Kreps, Haas, and half-a-dozen others. Everybody was in high spirits, and Cranston exuded a relaxed charm that I hadn't thought possible. Kreps made a point of sitting next to me, and while cutting into Vic's splendid lemon butter veal, I discovered why. He spoke very softly, in the conspiratorial tone he loved to affect. "Dick, we're moving fast on staffing. What job do you want on the Washington staff?"

I should have expected the question — virtually everybody who goes to work at a senior level in a campaign does so with an eye on a job if his man is elected — but the question took me quite by surprise. Kreps was looking at me intently. He had become my friend, there was no doubt that he was speaking for Cranston, and he wanted an answer. Certainly, I had planned to go to Washington on the wave of a Kennedy victory, but that was a very different scenario. Being a political appointee of a President was one thing; being a legislative aide to a freshman senator, no matter how senior the staff position, was much less seductive. I had developed a genuine affection for Cranston and thought he would do good things, but I couldn't foresee the rise to eminence as Democratic party whip that in a few years would carry his loyal staffers to positions of power and respect in the congressional apparatus. All he looked like at lunch was an amiable, hardworking, good man who would make few waves.

Beyond the fact that I didn't regard a move to Washington with Cranston as a particularly astute personal power play, there was the off-putting lack of style and flair not only in Cranston himself, but in the people around him. I could have gotten to enjoy Kreps despite his pomposity, but he was returning to law practice. Craggy Lu Haas, the only really blithe spirit in the bunch, would be running Cranston's L.A. office, and would not be around to drink with and exchange old war stories. The two people who would certainly be going with Cranston were competent political journeymen who, like the senator, would do good jobs but who, also like the senator, were boring as sin. I didn't know then that they would soon become recognized as the ablest administrative aide and best press aide in Washington. All I knew was that they wore polyester suits that glowed in the sunlight, with short-sleeved shirts underneath them, they had never seen a marijuana joint, they didn't go to discos or much of anyplace else after dark, and they apparently slept only with their wives. Even with a little bit of power in their hands, they seemed to me then to lack the instinct and the class for its proper enjoyment.

"Allyn," I said, "I can't tell you how flattered I am by the offer, but you know I really didn't go into the campaign to get a big job. I did it to help out a man I admire, whose politics I respect, and that's all there was to it. At this point in my life, I have too many other things going and, besides, the Washington money wouldn't be enough for me. But I'm sure you know that Alan can count on me for support and help of any other kind. I'm just not in a position to go to work for him."

Kreps had assumed that I was a political hanger-on with a great hunger for a big job. He was stunned. He said he was sorry and looked at me with a new respect. And I secretly relished a feeling of great freedom and satisfaction; I had matured from a chronic supplicant into an independent operator who could afford to turn down a job that other ambitious young men would have jumped at. I had no sense at all of having missed a very fast train.

As we left Trader Vic's I took Cranston aside and told him of my talk with Kreps and how much I regretted being unable to accept his flattering offer. He said he regretted it too. "It was a great campaign, Dick, and you did a wonderful job. I hope I'll be able to count on your continued support and help in other ways."

I assured him that he could count on me and I walked off alone down Cosmo Place, secure in the feeling that I now had a United States senator owing me. And, as Mel had predicted, it felt very good.

In January of 1969 Mel made good on his promise of a vice-presidency in his company, and told me to go down to the local Ford dealer and pick out a car. I had bought a Plymouth Barracuda a few months before and was thinking about picking out a convertible, but Mel astutely suggested that, since the company was paying for the car and none of the other officers had yet figured out what I was doing there other than being Mel's closest friend, it might be prudent to get something more conservative. Cost was no object, but appearance was. So I got a fully loaded station wagon, which made Arlene and the children happy.

Toward the end of the month, Mel put on a big dinner in Monterey for the company's officers, prime customers, and their wives. Arlene and I had driven there with Mel and Nina, and although the four of us were mildly drunk by the time the event was over, Mel insisted that it was too early to end the evening. We drove to Nina's new house in the nearby hills for music and more liquor. For the sake of corporate president-type appearances, Mel still maintained a separate address; they weren't married yet and, even in California, cohabitation among the unwed hadn't yet become a fashion in the better circles. But all his clothes were at Nina's house, as was his marijuana stash, and it was clear he'd moved in.

Mel put the Beatles on the stereo, poured us hefty drinks, and we all got a little drunker. Except for the raucous Carmel weekend, where serious talk had been impossible, Arlene had spent very little time around Mel, and he sensed that what she'd seen she didn't like. It was time for one of his maudlin monologues on the value of a few true friends amidst the hardness of life. He told Arlene of the depth of our friendship, of my great value to the company, and of all the triumphs that we were going to achieve together. He talked about Kennedy, and his eyes moistened when he reminisced about how he and I had met in that wonderful time. And he talked about how impressed he was with Arlene's beauty and intelligence. We would make a wonderful team, the four of us.

With the night wearing on, and Mel's scotch no longer adequate by itself as a fuel for his soaring sentiments, he went into the bedroom and fetched a huge bag of marijuana.

"It's time we turned on and loosened up," he said.

I was nervous. "Well, I don't know. It's getting late. Besides, Arlene's never smoked pot."

"So what," she said. "It's about time I did. And I can speak for myself."

Mel was beside himself with joy. "Oh that's beautiful, Arlene, just *beautiful*. I really love you," he slurred through a drunken grin, as he gave her a big hug and a kiss on the cheek.

73

It was "silly" pot, and before long Mel and Nina and I were off on a laughing jag, exploding in mirth at every uttered word, however inane. Arlene was sitting in a stony silence, and I could sense her slipping into the paranoia of somebody who has smoked pot but isn't on the communal wave length. I was laughing uncontrollably, even as I felt the anxiety build within me that Arlene's rigid face and angry eyes signaled an imminent catastrophe.

But suddenly the stern visage cracked and she erupted into almost hysterical laughter — at absolutely nothing at all. She rocked back and forth, tears streaming down her white face, and I was more afraid of her senseless mirth than I had been of her silence.

In a few minutes our hysteria vanished as quickly as it had come and the four of us sat in silence, listening to the music and looking out at the black bay and the distant lights of the city. Mel slipped his arm around Nina's shoulder. The pot had smoothed out our brains, we were mellow, and he wanted to share with us a wonderful gift. The hand at the end of his long right arm dangled languidly down to Nina's breast, and gently massaged the silk that enclosed it. "Hey, Richard, Arlene, don't you think Nina has great tits? Well, I guess you really can't tell, so I want you to look at this." And, bringing his other hand around the front of her, he unbuttoned her blouse, pulled one side of it off her, and cupped a single breast in both hands. He surveyed it briefly, as though examining a fruit for ripeness, then lowered his head and sucked it into his mouth. Nina feigned shock, then smiled and moaned a little as she put a hand on the back of his head and pressed it closer.

Arlene and I were quite dumbfounded. I allowed as how Nina did indeed have beautiful tits, and shortly I thanked Mel for the wonderful evening and we took our leave. Arlene and I drove on in silence up U.S. 101 to the city, each of us engrossed in our own contemplation of a

74

strange night. I had no hint of Arlene's feelings; but the pot and the spectacle of Nina's publicly consumed breast had left me aroused. For the first time in months, I felt like making love.

The sixties were running out. A large dream had died, but new ones were rising in its place. That decade left me with a larger appetite for life; it also left me with a paradox. It was strange to feel so full of life's bounties, and at the same time sense within me the growing of a void.

3
Sated Appetites

T HE sixties left me with a robust appetite for every
pleasure offered by the new, openly proclaimed hedonism, and with a mind liberated from the vestiges of
Puritan warnings. I was "free." But those years also left
me without even the pretense of a purpose larger than
myself. If the God that, as a child, I had been taught to
fear was finally and mercifully dead, then so were the
"great causes" of my adulthood. As the next decade began,
my friends and I — and hundreds of thousands of others
unknown to us but united by the common bond of lost
illusions — found ourselves alone together in a privileged
crowd that bubbled with wealth, appetite, and disen-
chantment. We had neither old roots nor new purposes.

It was a time that abounded with wizards full of insights
about the true path to fruition of the human potential.
With the sudden deflation of the social conscience of the
sixties, the great new truth — the "real" one — was conjured by the oracles of salvation. The flowering of the
individual was not to be found in engagement in "causes,"
or even in loyalties to once-solemn personal relationships — they, we learned, were grounded in saccharine,
self-defeating sentimentality — but in the uninhibited search
for new highs of private pleasure, private enlightenment,

private enrichment, and private joy. Our quest turned to the sating of heightened appetites and the finding of ourselves in selfishness.

The wisdom of the time coincided with my need. I was pushing forty, a willing candidate for middle-aged baptism into the new gospel of salvation through self-indulgence. Masquerades of do-goodism were no longer necessary. I could strive for power, position, and money openly. The pursuit of self was justified by its own delights.

I became an enthusiastic front-runner in the chase. My self-conscious idealism that, in the sixties, had put a noble if naïve face on my power craving, had faded, and my heroes had died, but the appetite for the good life learned in the sixties had survived. Although my adventures in the sixties hadn't led to a pinnacle of political office, they did leave me with two invaluable assets — a new political sophistication and a set of smart, ambitious friends, themselves propelled toward places of influence that would serve me well.

Shortly after Cranston took his oath of office, he telephoned to ask that I take a two-week leave of absence from my work and come to Washington to help him write a technically difficult article on a peacetime reconversion of the U.S. economy after the Vietnam war. All of our previous time together had been spent in the pressure cooker of an election campaign, and we hadn't really gotten to know each other; this was a splendid chance to remedy that. It was also a chance to increase his indebtedness to me. I figured that he owed me; I had played a significant role in his election and had declined his offer of a top job on his Senate staff. The campaign work had been well compensated, but this was different — a respected private sector professional graciously proffering his talents without pay for the public good at the request of a United States senator. It was the stuff from which glittering careers were fashioned.

By 1970 I was ready to take a major step in my life. My well-paid but ill-defined job had saved me from financial disaster and I had been grateful for it. And as Mel's influence as a political financial angel had continued to grow among California Democrats, so had my own reputation. Wealthy establishment Democrats treated me as a real "comer"; maître d's at La Bourgogne and Trader Vic's were newly deferential; and the sleek, discriminating women who frequented Pacific Heights' elite cocktail parties and the city's toniest restaurant bars proffered approving glances, then laughter over shared drinks, then invitations. Nonetheless, Mel's patronage had had its downside; he was a patron who just couldn't help patronizing, and that had become an increasingly bothersome thorn. Even though he had been generous to a fault, I knew I could earn a lot more money and harvest a lot more prestige out from under his possessive, if loving, wing. Feeling sure of my professional skills and social sophistication, and greatly strengthened by my valued contacts, I decided to return to the government affairs consulting business that I had ventured into for a year before I joined Kennedy. Only this time, it would be as my own boss — a seasoned, well-connected professional with considerable political clout.

Predictably, Mel took my announcement as a personal hurt. But equally predictably, he gave me his moral support, a loan, and my first small consulting job. Within a year I enlisted Cranston's support in my pursuit of the much-sought-after contract for appointment as the Golden Gate Bridge, Highway and Transportation District's federal lobbyist, and eventually parlayed the connection into a prestigious consulting business. By the middle of the seventies, I had gotten the district some forty million federal dollars for a bus and ferryboat system that the old political pros had said the feds would never pay for; and subsequently I would get the feds to pay another forty million for a new deck on the bridge, by getting my friends in Congress to amend the Federal Highway Act to afford my client favored treatment.

My reputation for successful lobbying spread quickly and far. My public agency clients soon included the Port of San Francisco, the Delaware River Port Authority, Marin County, the city of Honolulu, the state of Hawaii, Lake Tahoe's bi-state regional government, and the city of Detroit. I became an expert in development economics, and soon dollars were filling my pockets not only from government clients, but from major private developers as well.

My luxurious condominium on Tahoe's North Shore announced my achievements to that part of the San Francisco world that counted, and my regular patronage of the Madison Hotel in Washington told my eastern friends how sweet my life had gotten. I had become virtually a commuter between San Francisco and Washington, and the elegant and exclusive Madison had become my second home. When I arrived, the doorman and bell captain addressed me by name and the desk clerks never asked for a credit card imprint.

The Washington trips in those years were the best of times. I lived lavishly on unlimited expense accounts, and knew the menus at Sans Souci and Rive Gauche and Jacqueline's almost by heart. NBC had lifted Tom Brokaw from its Los Angeles affiliate and made him its White House correspondent, and he and his wife, Meredith, ever warm and loyal, always went out of their way to leaven my visits with the company of Washington's best and brightest. Each trip also included the ritual dinner with Sally Quinn. After Kennedy's assassination, Sally had returned to Washington emotionally battered, broke, and, along with the rest of us, dismayed by the ugly wreckage of suddenly shattered ambitions. But Sally was nothing if not resilient, and her place in the sun wasn't going to be denied by an assassin or anybody else; if she couldn't get there one way she'd do it another. In her early twenties, and without a column inch of journalistic experience, she had waltzed into the office of *Washington Post* editor Ben Bradlee, announced herself as a future star, and, astonishingly, landed a plum of a job writing personality feature stories and political gossip for the Style section.

Within a few months Sally had indeed become a star, if not quite an object of universal affection. As a writer, she was an apprentice then, but other talents more than compensated for her lack of journalistic experience. She had astounding gall, which, coupled with her nervy charm, got her access to the kinds of high-octane interviews that ordinarily could be managed only by the true titans of the media. She interviewed and deflated the façades of everybody from national security advisers to Iranian ambassadors to congressional powerhouses. She was smart and disarming, shrewdly fashioning questions that would unlock inhibitions and elicit ostensibly innocuous answers that, in fact, set the enamored victim up to be blithely led down the path of unintended self-revelation to ultimate public embarrassment.

The mystery of it all was that everyone loved being interviewed by Sally Quinn, although time and again they had seen her prior subjects savaged by her sure instinct for an Achilles' heel. And indeed they seemed to relish their *own* embarrassment in print even while they shouted obligatory rage at their "unfair" treatment.

Sally's company, in and of itself, was always a delight; but, in those days, her eminence in the town was a fine thing for me. She and Bradlee hadn't fallen in love and married yet, but she was getting to be enough of a personage in her own right to flavor my Washington trips with a cachet of influence and incipient power. Our dinners were always filled with inside gossip, ribald hilarity, and much good humor. They were special times. She wore her growing notoriety easily and without pretense. We joked about my unceasing efforts to bed her, and explored the elusive reasons for the repeated failures thereof with the feigned seriousness of philosophic inquiry. In our days of Robert Kennedy's California campaign, she had given me the come-on. But, as I slowly realized, it was only a strategy for getting a lift home across the bridge, where invariably a headache materialized. We talked about Kennedy and the old days, and about power and the future, and we became the truest of friends.

Sally and the Brokaws were such good comrades. When Arlene and I at last separated, thereby making the end of our long-failed marriage public and precipitating even more frequent trips east, they became my dedicated Washington social secretaries. There were the Friday meetings of the exclusive luncheon club at the Carlton, where I heard the great pontificate, and there was tennis with Richard Holbrook, the enfant terrible who was taking on the foreign policy establishment over its Asian policy and who later would become a major force in the State Department. Dates were arranged with Connie Chung and Leslie Stahl, neither of them quite national media stars yet, but, I was assured, both on their way there. Sally fixed me up with Barbara Howar, for a while Washington's premier political hostess; we became great friends for a time and I learned even more about *inside* Washington. I was also introduced to Doris Kearns, who had been Lyndon Johnson's confidante; it was gratifying to date the bright, well-connected young woman who later would write an intimate biography of LBJ and become a Harvard professor and marry Richard Goodwin, who had gotten famous working for JFK.

By the midseventies, I was well launched toward that envisioned earthly paradise of money and power that had long dominated my dreams. I loved the money I was making and the august company I was keeping, and back in San Francisco I was liking more and more the drug that made my rich life seem even richer, that pacified lingering anxieties and that was the fashionable symbol of my new success.

My lovely, feisty Melanie was a symbol of that success too, and the loss of her, while not quite a catastrophe, was hard to take. Melanie went her own way a couple of months after our tennis and cocaine adventure together in the summer of 1976. I had known that her departure was inevitable; she was very young and would soon be out of Stanford and she had her own worlds to conquer. But my realistic anticipation of her eventual flight hadn't made the actual event any easier for me. Melanie had taken off at a most unpropitious time, just when my negotiations with Arlene over a divorce settlement were getting dicey, and when I was also quarreling over money with my partner in the consulting business. She had occupied an important place in my bed, my social life, and my ego, and I had become accustomed to a fast sublimation of my problems in a woman's ready embrace. Now there was a large vacuum that had to be filled as soon as possible with some other sources of conveniently available sex and instant psychic reassurance.

I soon discovered that cocaine was just the right medicine. In the weeks after Mel had introduced me to the drug's wonders at the memorable tennis tournament, I had located a supplier of my own, and Melanie and I had enjoyed it through many long weekend nights, in the restaurants and discotheques, and at my apartment before and after making love. After she left in the autumn of 1976, I bought a lot more cocaine to fill the void and cure the gloom. During the late nights when I was alone in my bay view apartment, with only Vivaldi to keep me company, it mixed nicely with the Jack Daniels to conjure up feelings of lovableness and power, and to put the nagging problems of my daily business in their proper perspective. When the need for a woman couldn't be ignored, it fortified my charm and resolve for the ritual mating dance in the chic pickup bars at Perry's, Le Central, and MacArthur Park. In 1976 in San Francisco, a hint that you were prepared to jack up the lovemaking with some shared cocaine nearly always assured your conquest of the desired lady. Without regard for class, jobs, or social positions, the women in the city's fashionable watering holes shared a common passion: they wouldn't think of jumping in your bed for money, but a little high-quality coke almost assured their enthusiasm.

My drug played a central role in the sealing of my relationship with Melanie's replacement. I met Barbara at an opening in an avant-garde gallery and we took to each other right away. I had tired of my renewed body hustling in bars; and she, a self-proclaimed liberated and ambitious woman, was trying to cope with the blatant advances of her boss, a computer titan who increasingly was suggesting that her future in business would be at least as dependent on her performance in bed as on her office work. On the surface a woman who made much of her competence in life, she was in fact far less assured than she seemed and had an urgent need for a reassuring lover who didn't also pay her salary. If not a mesmerizing beauty, she was coolly attractive — an effect enhanced by the tailored suits she wore as declarations of serious, ungirlish purpose.

Barbara had discovered cocaine herself quite independently. After our first real date, she took me out to the house that she and her girlfriend rented, on a nice wooded piece of land in the Berkeley hills, where we smoked some grass, drank some wine, and went into the hot tub that sat on a redwood deck under the stars. We had some cocaine and made love, and then had some more cocaine.

Only a week after we had met, I had begun to find her disappointing. Although no great specimen myself, I had always been preoccupied with a search for physical perfection in women, and I found Barbara wanting on several

83

counts. And she made constant references to her purported 145 IQ, endlessly talked about her rich Texas family and the stock and cash she had inherited from her parents, the value of which she always smilingly refused to disclose, and launched into long-winded speeches about her independence as a woman.

But the wonderful thing about the cocaine was that, when I had enough of it along with some wine and pot, all the blemishes of body and personality disappeared, our normally mechanical lovemaking became adequately erotic, and she became a beautiful creature from whom I could get love and suitably decorative companionship.

Our third night with each other we had a lot of cocaine and, with our thought processes finely tuned, decided that we should live together. The next night we had even more cocaine, and brilliant ideas about what we should do with our lives emerged with a stunning clarity.

Barbara hated her compromised situation at the office and wanted an immediate and dramatic change of life. I too felt in need of a change, but I wasn't sure quite what. The night we met I had told her that I had a novel in me and that, if I could ever find the time, my dream was to write it.

"I have a wonderful idea," she said after we each had five or six snorts of coke. "Why don't we take a year off from work and go live in your house in Tahoe? You can write your book. I have money of my own, so I'll pay half of the expenses."

"That's fantastic. Let's do it," I said. With a little help from the coke, confusions were untangled, uncertainties were disarmed, analytical powers were sharpened, and I was emboldened to take courageous steps. The speed of it all was amazing. The next day I packed my personal effects in some cartons and walked away from a prospering but increasingly bothersome consulting business. I had spent eight hardworking years building the practice and establishing my professional reputation, but I left without a touch of regret. With a single shrug I unburdened myself of the heavy load of daily details and mundane frustrations, and the feeling of release was so euphoric that I didn't even bother to negotiate a cash settlement for my share of the business. I considered myself blessed simply to be escaping, without complications, into new horizons. I went to the bank and refinanced my condominium, and got thirty thousand dollars in cash. The transaction increased my mortgage from eighty to a hundred and ten thousand, but I was sure I could handle it. Cocaine had been a fantastic recreation; now I discovered how valuable it could be in helping with life's big decisions.

The year, which passed all too quickly, didn't work out as planned. Barbara and I played tennis and skied a lot, cavorted in Tahoe's livelier saloons, dined frequently on French cuisine at Le Petit Pier, acquired rich suntans, and learned to lie to each other. But the great novel did not get written. There was no book, not even a rough imitation of one, only a batch of repetitive, self-indulgent pontifications produced by a cocaine-liberated imagination.

As the project's formlessness became increasingly frustrating, the need for mind-clarifying became more frequent. Tennis — two or three times a day — was good for the mind as well as the body. Nightly dancing and drinking at Squaw Valley was great therapy. And cocaine and pot fueled the escalated schedule of careless lovemaking that now filled my expanded time.

Before the year was out, my thirty thousand dollars was gone. There had been a "misunderstanding," Barbara said, about her agreement to pay half of our living costs. She said she had meant only half of the grocery and entertainment costs, and the same amount for rent that she had paid when living with her roommate — a couple of hundred dollars a month, not half of the condominium costs. She was liberated, but not *that* liberated. With the increased mortgage payments, I had had to pay fourteen hundred dollars a month on the condo alone. And my initial twenty-five-hundred-dollar cocaine inventory had vanished in less than a month. But there had been no need to worry about the drug's availability at Tahoe; it was everywhere, and I had spent thousands — I had no idea how *many* thousands — to keep our spirits elevated.

By the early spring of 1978, I was flat broke and I didn't even have money for the cocaine that, in an instant, could have dispelled the gloom and made life bright again. Barbara and I were at each other all the time. She was feeling guilty about not working, and I was feeling guilty about having abandoned my profession and failing to produce a book. We had started the lies months earlier — lies about who had money and how much, lies about our understanding of the terms of our arrangement, and, most of all, lies about cocaine. Lies about who had had how much the night before, and who had how much hidden away in a cupboard or closet or shoe bag. Now, with all the coke gone, our views of each other became badly distorted. I found her imperfections more offensive than ever, and she repeatedly told me that I was looking old around the eyes. Finally, we quit making love.

I had to sell the condominium, my last asset, at no profit. The only thing I had acquired during my year of romance and literary pretense — apart from the beginning of a new affinity for debt — was a lusty taste for cocaine. And a taste for cocaine without money was a sour taste indeed.

Barbara and I began packing for the trip back to San Francisco, without the slightest idea of what we were going to do when we got there. I had reached a point in my life where there seemed no place to go but off a cliff.

I was saved by a telephone call from Lowell Edington, a power in Napa County politics and a controlling force on the Golden Gate Bridge District's board of directors.

As a result of my lobbying work for the district over some seven years, he had become a close friend, admirer, and patron. Lowell said that the district desperately needed me again to do some economic analyses and political work to get a transit tax approved, as well as to do some more lobbying in Washington. I was being offered a five-thousand-dollar retainer up front on a contract that, although initially for fifty thousand, could be amended for more. At my darkest moment, my talents and professional reputation had been remembered.

Barbara and I got to San Francisco as quickly as we could. Encouraged by my recouped fortunes, she sold some stock and threw four thousand dollars into a financial pot that we would use to get reestablished. The first thing we did was rent a sensational house with a glass wall on a Sausalito hill, with an unimpeded view of the bay. The second thing we did was buy some cocaine and treat ourselves to a heavy celebratory dose. With our disordered psyches now straightened out, we fell in love again for a while.

The rest of 1978 was a generally up year, and it flew by with a minimum of problems. Barbara got herself a prestige job with a blue chip firm and, with her much-advertised IQ now productively displayed among the moguls of Montgomery Street, felt quite good about herself for a time. I immersed myself in work and local politics, traveled frequently on invigorating business trips to Washington, and got my life back together.

It was true that I had had to rethink my use of cocaine. Abandoning the drug was out of the question; the extraordinary benefits it offered foreclosed such a drastic step. On the other hand, there was no denying the drug's judgment-distorting role in the Tahoe fiasco that had nearly finished me. And I had spent huge amounts that I couldn't afford for cocaine. The trick was to use it for the right purposes in the right situations, and to avoid the pitfalls.

Balance, that was the thing. The problem, I figured out, was not that I had spent too much per se for the drug, but that I had spent the money when I didn't have any income to replace it. But that was in the past. I was *back*. And I felt good.

By the end of 1978, I had three solid clients that I expected to pay me a total of about $150,000 in annual billings — a modest amount compared to the incomes of some of my friends, but certainly marginally sufficient to maintain me as an habitué of the elegant boutiques, restaurants, and watering holes that were the *sine qua non* of having "made it." I forgot my ideas of balancing my intake of cocaine. I was taking more than ever, using it in increasing amounts for work as well as play. There was no apparent physical damage and cocaine was opening doors for me. There was money enough not only to sustain my own habit, but to finance ever larger purchases to reciprocate my much wealthier friends' past years of generosity, and to establish myself as a fully credentialed member of their golden circle. My new generosity as a cocaine source greatly enhanced my already considerable reputation as a good guy. The warm solicitude that greeted me now upon my arrivals at the exclusive little bistro that served as headquarters for San Francisco's hip political and entrepreneurial crowd of rich cocaine aficionados was truly remarkable; my now endless and always shared cocaine supply irrefutably established that I had arrived. The tables I now got at the bistro were invariably superior.

With my prosperity revived, Barbara and I decided to greet 1979 with a New Year's Eve party. It would be a chance to return years of hospitality provided by my rich friends, to exchange affections in the warmth of the holiday glow, and to let it be known that I was no longer on the dole. A modest entertainment would never do. It would have to be lavish, it would have to be elegant, and it would have to be pricey. Simplicity could be misunderstood.

To set the tone, the gentlemen's dress would be black tie, which in turn would guarantee the ladies' adornment in their most elegant gowns. Among our class of newly prosperous, immigrant San Franciscans (as distinguished from the third- and fourth-generation legatees of old, established fortunes), casual elegance was the norm; formal dress was virtually nonexistent except at the opera (which we didn't attend) or the thousand-dollar-a-plate political fund-raising dinners that the nouveaux riches periodically graced to demonstrate their identification, as good Democrats, with the cause of the poor. It was virtually unheard of to wear formal attire at home, particularly in the ultra-hip ambiance of the Sausalito hills, where Ralph Lauren shirts and designer jeans were much more reflective of laid-back sensibilities and much easier to shed in the after-dinner rush to assorted hot tubs and other entertainments. Our guests greeted our announcement of an upscale party with great enthusiasm. Everyone would be so *handsome*. So *elegant*. So *right*. As though we were actually in New York or London.

There would be twelve of us. We would do a buffet — but *elegantly*. Of course. Dozens of freshly shucked oysters and plump shrimp, caviar, five pounds of fresh cracked crab, manicotti and the city's most delicate prosciutto. The wines would be perfect — an assortment of the finest Bordeaux, some exquisite Montrachet, and, for the New Year, Cristal champagne, the costliest bubbly that France had to offer. Of course. The cost of food and wine for the twelve of us (without catering, which we casually explained was not a matter of cost, but because "we just *so* enjoy doing these things ourselves; it's so much fun") would be just under two thousand dollars. For me, a lot. But then, what are friends for?

With the first arrivals, it was plain that we had concocted

a night to remember. Each couple crossed our threshold aglow with beauty, charm, anticipation, and the thrill of being delightfully full of themselves — the men's tanned faces even handsomer than usual by virtue of the stark black and white tuxedos (in our group the faces were *always* tanned, even in midwinter); the women surpassingly gorgeous in their clinging designer silks and satins. Wilkes Bashford — San Francisco's preeminent purveyor of outlandishly priced, but incontestably *au courant,* clothes to the city's rich hip set — had clearly had a very good day. None of our group, except one of the women (who somehow had managed to survive despite her occasional flashes of independence), would think of appearing at a "significant event" attired in anything that didn't have the unmistakable Wilkes look. But tonight even the tuxedos were clearly identifiable as the merchandise of the master — at a thousand dollars a shot. All the evidence was in: the people who mattered had judged our party a *significant event.*

There was more to this gathering than a display of ostentatious tastes. While each of us, in our separate but frequently converging ways, had embarked on single-minded odysseys to acquire fame and fortune and to squander both as fast and frequently as possible, we had still retained the capacity to care deeply about each other. Strangely, with all our growing narcissism, our emotional bonds were drawn more tightly now than ever. We felt ourselves a special group that had been joined insolubly together in special times, a group apart; and in our apartness we loved ourselves and each other.

Michael and Alice were the first to arrive; among other virtues, they were never late. Now in his midforties, Michael, in addition to drawing a six-figure salary as a corporate executive, had proved to have a golden touch in the stock market. He was a millionaire several times over, and since the Kennedy campaign had become a financial power in Democratic politics. He came from a dirt poor family in Appalachia, had worked his way through the world's best universities, and acquired an extraordinary charm, cultivation, and taste for things civilized. He had a rich spirit, an unambiguous zest for life taken at face value, without a hidden agenda, and was smarter at more levels than anybody else I've ever known. Michael understood me completely, and I him. We took each other for what we were — no questions asked. Our unspoken understanding of each other's weaknesses, coupled with unconditional acceptance, was magic and special.

Alice was his second wife. I had met Michael when he was still living with his first one, sort of. I had seen him through, and covered for, his infidelities; when the separation finally became clean, we accompanied each other in open revelries with a series of girlfriends — some "serious" and others the playthings of the moment. And as the breakup of my own marriage followed his, he had seen me through the tough parts. Michael and Alice had met a couple of years before and had instantly fallen in love. She had, as they say, been around. Sixteen years younger than Michael, she was of the openly "liberated" generation, and had spent her early twenties traveling in the fast lane along the Atlantic seaboard, accumulating experiences that Michael in his wildest fantasies could only dream about.

When Michael had first brought Alice into San Francisco for his friends' approval, there was much whispering, tsk-tsking, and shaking of heads. Poor Michael had to be warned off this folly of a relationship that he seemed intent on pursuing to a serious conclusion. Who was this girl, anyway? A bit brash, obviously without much of a background. She apparently had had some college and could converse with some sparkle and intelligence socially, but she had too much vivacity for comfort, and an openness that was decidedly uncool. Nobody knew anything about her or where she had come from. And everybody feared that Michael didn't know much about her either. Since Michael was by now rich and this assertive little snip obviously didn't have a sou, it was clear to all that this was a gold digger on the make and Michael had better watch out. So the ladies in the group took it upon themselves to defend Michael's true interests by cutting poor little Alice up into as many delicately sliced pieces as possible at every opportunity. And Mel had been quick to join the ladies in the carving. When Mel went after somebody who disturbed his view of the way the world ought to be, he did so with the vengeance of a fishwife. He and his wife, Nina, were, at least in that regard, a perfect match; she shared Mel's instinct for the human jugular, but pursued it with more subtlety. Mel assaulted the victim with a meat ax while Nina specialized in the nuances of the forked tongue.

Our little family had lived its incestuous fantasies of self-importance for so long that *anybody* presuming to intrude herself into the life of one of the principals would have been in for a very hard time. And that was particularly true when the pursued was Michael. With his looks, his charm, his self-made wealth, and his joie de vivre, he was everybody's hero. Even Mel really wanted to be Michael when he grew up. Each of us had had our own piece of Michael, and Mel and Nina weren't about to share theirs. But Alice had guts and stood her ground. She wanted Michael's friends' approval; but if, in their absurd pretensions, they were too emotionally constipated to give it, to hell with them. She would have what she would have. Michael needed her in his life.

After a year or so together they had resolved to marry, and did. As her tough integrity and simple charm had become apparent, and it had become clear that Michael's resolve could not be shaken, one and all had — with much self-congratulation — accepted her into the golden circle; a fact that impressed the bestowers of approval much more than it did her. Alice, with her sense of self, could have done quite nicely without it, thank you. In fact, she turned out to be the lady of them all.

Tough but honestly sentimental, taking little note of her enemies, she had taken Michael in tow and, although he was beyond the reach of total domestication, had tamed him into a responsible and even slightly fearful husband — fearful only because he didn't want to lose her. In Alice, quite apart from Michael, I now had another great and loyal friend.

They greeted me the night of the party with the usual openers. First Alice's whispered aside: "What an asshole he is. I'm sorry, I'm in a bitchy mood, but he's impossible to live with." Followed by Michael's "Christ, I've really got to be careful tonight. She's really pissed. Tell you about it later. Have you got any coke?" Whereupon both proceeded to saunter into the house, their domestic spat over and very much in love.

Mel and Nina arrived next. He with the lanky body and loose shuffle that seemed the essence of casual hipness, the slight, knowing smile, and the big bear hug and kiss on the cheek. (The more despairing his life at home, the greater Mel's displays of love toward his friends had become.) She, as always, was dressed for show, but her once-gentle face was puffy, her hair dull, her eyes glassy, and the hollows under them a poorly covered-up purple. The couple's holidays had obviously been more festive than ever — replete with nightly drug, booze, and sex parties, inevitably followed by violent fights and efforts to maintain the pretense of respectability and holiday happiness for the children from their previous marriages. They indulged in endless accusations and recriminations having to do with the alarmingly rapid outflow of money. Mel complained of the cost of educating her kids; Nina blamed his cocaine habit, although her drug compulsion was as great as his. Mel's negotiations to sell his company to some foreign investors, to make the quick hit on the stock market that would bail him and Nina out of the consequences of their excesses, had been going on for two years. It all took a lot of negative energy, and they looked it. But, for a few hours at least, they would overcome the festering pathos of their lives. As Mel hugged me and kissed me on the cheek, he mumbled, "Richard, how about a little coke?"

The core group had assembled — Michael, Mel, their wives, and me. There were others to arrive whom, in varying degrees, we had taken into the periphery of our enchanted world. All were fondly regarded, although none could really invade the core. But these others had their roles, and neither our party scene nor a picture of my life then would be complete without them.

There were Kenneth and Diana, rich and beautiful — almost indecently so. Although he was part-owner of an art gallery to create the appearance that, like everybody else, he had to work for a living, Kenneth was supported in great luxury by inherited wealth. He and golden-haired Diana — by unanimous agreement, the most authentically gorgeous woman any of us had ever seen — devoted their time and energy primarily to keeping their bodies perfect, and to the growth of self-knowledge. They ran ten miles a day in designer jogging suits, explored the depths of their psyches under the guidance of the best Jungian analysts, and meditated a lot. In their physical perfection, and in the benign goodwill of their breathless reports on the mysteries of the collective unconscious, they were like a couple from another planet. They were beautiful, inoffensive, and caring, and we always delighted in their company without taking them too seriously. Kenneth and Diana enjoyed a few toots of cocaine now and then socially, but the drug wasn't as important to them as it was to the rest of us. Kenneth's consciousness was still wrapped up in the psychic romance of the sixties, and consciousness-raising was his thing. He would say things like, "Richard,

I wish you would take an acid trip with me sometime and see the cosmos."

George and Joanne were barely thirty, years younger than the rest of us, but they fitted in nicely. Intensely ambitious for money and social position, they found our group's attraction — particularly Michael's — irresistible. George was slender and handsome, very bright, and full of goodwill; and Joanne, although she was a bit too pushy, was a genuine young beauty with fetching blond hair arranged in expensive wild disarray; she had a small waist, slender legs, and firm breasts, and all of this was invariably displayed in Wilkes Bashford's costliest outfits. Our quick acceptance of George and Joanne as social playmates was motivated by more than their beauty and charm. George was going to law school nights and worked during the day. But their coke business, which Joanne managed, was their big source of income. Most drug dealers were seedy, shifty types dwelling on the margin of society. You always felt a little dirty doing business with them, and a little nervous. To have a supply of high-quality coke available at a moment's notice from beautiful people of your own social class was a wonderful thing.

Kenneth's young stockbroker and his wife were the last to arrive. They had been high school sweethearts in Idaho farm country, and after college they had married and found their way to the big city. Through their friendship with Ken and Diana, they had gotten their first taste of big money and the sweet life. They were compulsive spenders and heavy cocaine users. Nobody liked the wife much — the airs she had started affecting were too obvious — but Jimmy was a delight. He was basically an uncomplicated farmboy mesmerized by the bright lights. He had made himself a wine expert, and it was very amusing to see him roll some expensive Bordeaux around in his mouth, furrow his brow and pucker his lips for a few minutes of quiet contemplation, help himself to a couple of snorts of cocaine in the manner of a true sophisticate, and then ultimately pronounce his connoisseur's judgment on the wine in accents straight out of potato country.

The night was cool and clear. From our house perched on a Sausalito hill less than a mile from the northern bank of the Golden Gate, we looked through a ten-foot-high wall of glass at a million lights twinkling in the hills of Berkeley across the bay to the east. Southward, the skyline of San Francisco delicately raised itself above the blackness of the water, announcing its presence by a million more lights. Below our wall of glass a dozen or so herring boats — early arrivals from as far away as Seattle — slowly plied the waters. When I opened the wall, the only sounds were the lapping of the water on the rocks below, the laughter and profane shouts that passed from boat to boat, the occasional splash of a beer bottle tossed into the bay, and the caws of gulls.

That night, my friends and I *identified* with the fishermen in the boats below. We talked about how much fun it would be to go down and party with them or to invite them to join us for our holiday celebration. It didn't occur to us that they would probably greet us with the disdain that the workmen of the world reserve for the soft and privileged; or that, if they came to my house, they would spoil the occasion by trudging over my white, deep-pile carpets with rubber boots rank with the remnants of fish guts. Of course, it didn't occur to us that, in our enthusiasm for a night of cultural exchange with the "salt of the earth," we were indulging the same quaint urges of privilege that, twenty years before, had impelled those of us who had been schooled in New England to take our girlfriends down to Harlem — in the days when rich whities and their money were welcome there — to listen to jazz and blues and graciously slum in the name of liberal enlightenment.

It was not a night for examining attitudes deeply. The

world was one, and we were at one with the world. In any case, the fishermen were there and we were here, in love with ourselves and each other, our palates piqued by a splendid array of delicate food and exquisite wines arranged on a great table of Italian glass.

As the eating began to wind down, I set an onyx slab on a large, round coffee table and told my guests to gather round. They did so without having to be asked twice, having correctly surmised that the bewitching hour had at last arrived. When the evening had begun, and most of my guests had, as soon as their feet were through the door, inquired as to the availability of "a little coke" (knowing full well, of course, that there would not be a little, but a lot), I had politely demurred, explaining that that happy hour would come, but not quite yet. Tonight was going to be different. For a change, we weren't going to start snorting with the first hello (at least not publicly) and ruin our ability to enjoy the food that I had so painstakingly prepared; no, we would delight in a short period of discipline, postpone the drug for a while, and enjoy a time of undistorted appreciation of good food, mellow music, and each other. Everyone understood and none protested — a response made easier by the fact that, as I knew (and as they knew I knew), they all carried their own surreptitious stash, which would see them privately through the hours until the host saw fit to produce the communal treasure. This had two virtues. It enabled the host to preserve his big supply until those late-night hours when, after too much food and wine and the onset of fatigue, serious snorting became important. (If the drug were offered earlier, it would be gone within the hour, the nature of coke and its devotees being that, however much is put out in a communal setting, it will *all* be consumed as rapidly and compulsively as is humanly possible.) The second advantage of the game of "Oh, you do have some coke but want to save it until later; that's cool" is that everyone could then proceed through the early hours in secret consumption of his or her own supply while pretending abstinence and not having to share the costly stuff with anybody else, which was the host's responsibility. It was a system that made everybody comfortable.

So, throughout the early evening, the bathroom had been continually occupied, as my guests — and I — rotated turns of tiny "secret" toots to keep us going until the big event. And, however silly the institutional hypocrisy of it all, in this way consumption was kept modest for a while, personalities were kept intact a bit longer, and everybody was able to partake at his own rhythm of the drug that, for us all, had become the essential accoutrement of our social selves. For a year now, neither Michael, Mel, nor I — nor our women — had once gone out after the sun went down without first getting jacked up with cocaine, and without using it throughout those endless nights to keep ourselves electric. Not once. We, who had been jovial comrades for some eight years before we discovered the drug, now were not sure that we could even talk interestingly to each other without it. And we were not of a mind to try.

But the hours of pretense were past; the time was at hand for the night's serious business. From the pocket of my dinner jacket I produced a plastic bag full of a half-ounce of cocaine acquired earlier in the day, in a frantic last-minute rush, from Joanne, who, having maintained a discreet silence through the earlier evening, now benignly smiled with that disquieting condescension of all dope dealers — whether of high society or of the street — who know that their friends' (clients') lives depend on them. Cost, thirteen hundred dollars — which did not include the other half-ounce at an additional thirteen hundred dollars that I had acquired that day and secretly stashed away for my own future happiness.

While lips smiled and eyes sparkled, I dumped a healthy mound on the onyx slab and, with a razor blade, chopped the grains more finely, formed a new pile of the powder, and divided it into long, thin lines. I handed Mel a small gold tube and watched him proceed to snort what he knew was twice his allotted share up his large and most efficient nose. (None of us minded that Mel always took more than his share; his coke greed was accepted as part of his charm. It would be another year before he paid the price suffered by many coke gluttons — a perforated septum, i.e., holes that the drug's acidity eats into the cartilage that separates the nostrils. Not wanting his nose to collapse — yet not wanting to give up the drug — he solved the dilemma by sucking the powder directly into his throat for a time until he temporarily lost his voice. With resignation, he finally went back to the nose — which apparently held up all right despite its internostril ventilation.) The onyx slab was passed from guest to guest, each of whom in turn inhaled deeply of the stuff, said something like "Oh, that *is* nice," and passed it on to the next guest. When the lines were gone, I dumped some more of the glistening powder and cut it into more lines. And so it went around the table on into the night. With the uplifting music of Christmas carols and occasional Bach playing softly in the background, the convocation was getting into the spirit of things.

Sometime in the late seventies, the liberal rich, and those who fancied themselves as rich without really being so, transformed cocaine from its function as merely a fun drug into a secular sacrament. In the long-ago days when Mel had given me my first snort, the required equipment was simplicity itself. If you were doing it on the run, in a telephone booth or toilet stall, all you needed was a little glass vial and a tiny stainless-steel spoon. If you were doing it with friends in the more gracious circumstances of your parlor, the preferred method was to dump the drug on a slick surface, usually a simple mirror, cut the lines with a mundane razor blade, and snort them up with a plastic straw.

Those two methods of tooting the stuff were uncomplicated and cheap: maybe five dollars for the complete kit. But, it had become the fashion among my friends and me — and indeed among everyone we played with from Nob Hill to Beverly Hills to Park Avenue — to employ elegant "designer" equipment in our ingestion of cocaine. If our image of the typical heroin shooter was that of a wasted failure sticking a rusty needle into his vein below the sleeve of a grimy T-shirt, our own passion was obviously of a much different order. Their drug was cheap and ours cost a lot; their mode of ingestion was crude and ours, delicately effete. The square, uptight guardians of middle-class boredom, who suggested that those distinctions were not mitigating differences, simply didn't know where things were at.

This was to be a big occasion, and I had figured out that, if the evening's possibilities were to be fully realized, the old, standard equipment simply wouldn't do. Hence, the one-foot-square, two-inch-thick slab of solid onyx that I had purchased that afternoon at Gumps to use as a serving tray. The razor blade that I used to cut the lines of cocaine was gold plated, manufactured specifically for the purpose. And, as with the blade, the "tooter" — the short, slender tube that was the vital link between nose and coke — was also plated with a glistening gold. These items had not been hard to find. For some time the most exclusive jewelry stores in Manhattan, San Francisco, and Beverly Hills had been openly displaying gold, sometimes jewel-inlaid, items that had no conceivable functions other than the carrying, serving, and snorting of cocaine. Business was particularly brisk at Christmastime. (Indeed, that very evening George had taken me aside to present me with a holiday gift that bespoke not only his love but, not incidentally, his appreciation for some twelve thousand dollars of my business during the year — a carved ivory vial to carry my coke in, with a tiny, delicately curved, matching ivory spoon. "Don't tell anybody where you got this," he whispered. "Not everyone is getting one.")

And so we sat side by side on the floor around the large, round glass coffee table. Chatting gaily, telling our inside jokes, bowing our heads over the onyx altar as it was passed to us, and snorting our cocaine. I had gradually become aware over the past year of a new quality in our drug-taking occasions. It was one kind of experience to snort the drug alone, with casual acquaintances, or while out on the town — sneaking a toot in this bathroom and that one, while moving gaily from bar to restaurant. It had become quite another thing when, as now was increasingly the case, we met as a group of close friends in the relaxed privacy of our homes, to snort and drink communally and talk endlessly through endless nights. Some new compelling chemistry was at work among us *as a group*, above and beyond the direct effects of the drug itself. I hadn't yet been able to define my feeling — that vague sense of a new dynamic in our collective lives, which for a year had been growing on me without my understanding it. Barely a week before, I had felt it most strongly at Mel and Nina's Christmas dinner, which had become an annual tradition for Michael and Alice, Kenneth and Diana, and me. But tonight, the air was thick with the sense of this strange yet beautiful something to which I could not give a name. Then, quite suddenly, I understood.

The drug was no longer merely our casual fun; nor our private vice to be privately dealt with. It had become the sacrament of our friendship, binding us together in the celebrations of our victories; and, when various pieces of our lives had come unglued, it had become the nostrum that magically re-created in our collective mind the illusion that all was well. The drug had become our ultimate validator, not only of ourselves to ourselves, but of each of us to the others, and of all of us as a collective entity to the outside world.

Virtually from the beginning of the friendship that Michael, Mel, and I had, we had needed each other; we had derived great joy from our shared lives and critical reinforcement in times of trouble. That old need of togetherness — perhaps always a little strange, even in the days of innocence — was now, in our mildly advancing years, even greater. We *had* to be together — a lot. To laugh, to drink, to congratulate ourselves, and — most of all — to pontificate until dawn about philosophy and values, and so reinforce ourselves in our persuasions, and in our belief that behind the façades of glamour and materialism there thrived the souls of the serious. We *had* to be together; but it had become impossible to be together without cocaine. Its use both freed our individual spirits for flights of internal fantasy and united us in a common passion. It had become the compulsion for our convocations — the glue that bonded us together. We had moved the drug to the center of our lives, where it had become as constant and real a companion for each of us as we were to each other.

The sudden chill of recognition passed quickly. My mind had been spinning fantasies — nonsense to be put aside. I had been using the drug for over two years now, and in earlier periods had taken it in far greater amounts than was now my custom. I understood the drug. I knew what it did and didn't do to me. Wasn't I functioning better in my work and with my friends than I had in a long time?

I shook off my spell of dark reveries, for it was my turn to treat myself to another snort — all the guests having been more than nicely served during the last few rounds. I inhaled a line deeply into each nostril, immediately felt the effect of the fresh cocaine mingling in my head and senses with the marijuana fumes I had put there minutes before — and embarked on a trip of both private and social joy. The coke gave me a great shot of vitality, an abundance of exciting new ideas to share, a heightened awareness of my surroundings, and fresh insights into the hearts and minds of all people. And the grass was the perfect partner. Most weed we got our hands on in those days had too much of a downer effect; it simply put you out or made you nervous. The good marijuana — and this was some of the best — heightened all the senses, transformed surroundings into a softly lit amusement park, and — most importantly — mellowed out the nervous agitation that invariably accompanied the heavy use of potent cocaine. This was an especially felicitous mix of weed and coke; I was intellectually charged, spiritually attuned, and every sense was alive and processing data with both unbelievable speed and aesthetic acuity.

The lights on our tall, lushly spreading Christmas tree suddenly blossomed in an array of voluptuous colors; and each bulb, now mysteriously energized by a force that made electricity seem but a transient convenience, seemed to pulsate — now expanding in size, now diminishing and then expanding again. And, with each pulsation, the oranges, blues, yellows, greens, and reds deepened in their richness, as though the bulbs had tapped into the nourishing sap of the branches from which they hung, which in turn were drinking of primal energy from the ground below. In each contraction and expansion it was as if I was seeing the very heartbeat of the earth's life.

The only other illumination came from the votive candles I had placed about the room on low tables and in the staggered recesses of modular bookcases and other wall shelves where — mixed in with books, small plants, and assorted *objets d'art* — their flickering flames cast dancing silhouettes. Alice and I were holding hands now, misty-eyed with the beauty and holiness of it all, wordlessly enjoying the communion of our platonic love. The coke and grass had worked their synergistic magic and, in a wonderful rush of tactility, I felt her hand's skin, flesh, sinew, and blood merge with my own. From the stereo speakers, the tones of "Adeste Fideles" flowed into the room with a richness only partly created by the choir's artistry; for, as with the perceptions of sight and touch, the drugs had awakened the aural sensors in my brain to new heights of awareness. The music came to me not only in the fullness of choral ensemble, but in every single component that comprised the song. I heard the choir; but, with it, I perceived each of its separate parts — every individual voice singing personally to me, and every note of every chord floating distinctly and separately into the room like a full balloon, where it danced with its myriad partners and then united with them again in a rush of reconciled harmony. On this last night of the season of the birth of the Christ, *we had come to chapel* — not your usual chapel, mind you; but a place where sensual gluttony could cohabit comfortably with feigned piety, and where we could indulge the illusion that, despite our sophistications, materialistic compulsions, and deliberately severed roots, our souls were still tapped into the spiritual nourishment of ancestral soil from which — as our emotional whims moved us in holy seasons — we could suck up intimations of God, Bethlehem, grandparents, and a simple world of belief long lost.

Each in our turn, we accepted the golden straw and reverently inhaled our elixir from its altar. It was not frankincense and myrrh. But it certainly would do.

To the uninitiated, this no doubt seems a strange description — hedonism and holiness all of a piece. I had learned early on that this was one of my drug's great miracles — to move me swiftly and more deeply into the emotional environment of the moment, to give me that rush of power and involvement to be what I was expected to be in context. During the Christmas season, I was supposed to be warm, giving, and holy, however fatigued and frustrated I might feel. With cocaine, my friends and I *became* all of those things. And we did not even have to take the trouble to go to church to feel that way. We were already there. The gold-plated cocaine tooter had replaced the silver chalice.

At midnight I poured champagne. We sang "Auld Lang Syne," cried, and kissed each other. By two in the morning, most of the guests had departed. Because it had been at least half an hour since I had put any cocaine out, it was logical for them to assume that none was left, so there really wasn't any large reason — despite the undoubted trueness of our shared affections — for them to hang around longer. They would now retire to their own homes and privately snort their own stashes through what remained of the night. My turning off the supply had had its desired effect; all that were left now were the members of the inner circle — Mel, Michael, myself, and our ladies. I briefly excused myself, quickly poured into a film canister four grams from the second half-ounce that I had hidden out of Barbara's reach in the pocket of an old suit, and returned to the favored few. The six of us sat around the table until the sky began to lighten, around six, snorting, smoking grass, talking deeply about life and how we really felt about one another. It had become a familiar pattern after a night of booze, pot, and coke. All inhibitions were gone, brains were reeling with great truths that just had to be shared, hearts were bursting with feelings, and six well-lubricated tongues were poised to launch the inevitable nonstop, free-form pronouncements that, floating on undammed streams of consciousness, would flood the room with wisdom.

As always, the cocaine made us loquacious and sometimes even eloquent; and, if the sequential arrangement of our sentences sometimes exhibited less than a logical symmetry, the defect went unnoticed since what we were now about was not dialogue but the simultaneous presentation of six very earnest monologues. As always with coke, our feelings of intellectual superiority and emotional clarity were extraordinary. And, in our certainty that cocaine had again blessed us with valuable new insights and revelations, we once again were able to sublimate those pestering voices of the conscience that whispered of debauchery.

The problem was that we had begun to repeat ourselves. The great truths we announced that night had, during the previous couple of years, been announced at least two-dozen other times on occasions that differed less in their insightful substance than in their locale and the attire of the congregation. That, and the fact that any words that were indeed important could have been said, without cocaine, in about fifteen minutes. But brevity was never the point of a cocaine session; the great thing was to use the drug to compress time and expand consciousness, to make ten hours of nonstop partying seem but an hour or two of wired, high-energy *involvement* — a swatch of blissfully distorted time in which neither boredom nor self-doubt nor loneliness had a place. Achievement of such a time/energy distortion is no small task. Cocaine had the effect of electrifying minds and oiling tongues, thereby releasing rivers of seamless chatter. Nothing fills time so fully, or makes it pass so quickly, as the unrelieved sound of one's own mesmerizing words, unleashed by the destruction of all inhibitions.

But our magic night, like all good things, had to end. Good-byes had to be said before the full light of day was upon us, revealing the rheumy eyes and collapsed faces that bespoke not enlightenment but self-abuse, not a quickening of the spirit but compulsive decadence. The shining hot-air balloon that had carried us through one more night of euphoric escape was deflating quickly and soon would thud back to earth. Reality was at hand. There were the obligatory hugs and kisses all around that always ended our sessions, and the tearful words of love and thanks for everyone's honest revelations of his inner self. Everyone said how much the night had meant, and then, feeling the first hints of the fatigue that for several days would cripple them as wives, husbands, and parents, our guests drove off to their respective places of repair and interim rehabilitation. Until next time.

Barbara and I sank into the huge, soft Italian sofa that had been the first of the unaffordable purchases I made after my year of exile to announce my economic and social resurrection. It was full daylight now, but the Christmas tree lights still glowed and a few candle flames still flickered. Unwashed dishes were piled up in the kitchen, and the house was rank with the smell of cigarette butts, drying crabmeat, and stale oysters. The house would stay that way for two days. But for now, no matter. We talked for a few minutes about how fantastic the night had been and congratulated ourselves on our good taste and elegant performances. I relit an expired joint of marijuana, took the smoke deeply into my lungs, had a couple of snorts of cocaine, and slipped my hand beneath Barbara's mauve silk blouse. A responsive nipple hardened; she took a couple of quick tokes of the grass and went for my crotch.

It was but a short slide to the floor, where, without preliminary gentle kisses or whispered endearments, we proceeded to make the kind of love that had become our custom. With our drug-besotted brains churning out myriad erotic fantasies, it was all ravenous mouths, licking tongues, and heaving flesh, with every cell of skin vibrantly alive to the touch and every orifice given its due. With the coke and grass, the sensuousness quickly transcended the identities of the lovers, and the result was the astounding knowledge of lust as pure abstraction.

While people truly in love sometimes use drugs for an extra sexual kick, I had found the beauty of the cocaine and pot mix (on high occasions perhaps leavened with a little hypnotic Quaalude) to be its ability to promote among the *un*loving sex that is at once gorgeous and *mindless*. There was no need for me to think about who I was or who she was, or why we were rutting about on a carpet redolent of spilled wine and dropped ashes. For me, Barbara's abandonment was a mirror image of my own autoerotic delights, and I suspected — but didn't care — that for her it must be the same. For me, she was faceless and could have been anybody, and I suspected — but didn't care — that for her it must be the same. Primal sex without the burden of affection transported me, in my utter separateness, into a world of personal power free from reciprocal responsibility. I felt that if either of us harbored a large sentiment toward the other, surely it was rooted in the appreciation that each of us had for the ready availability of a reasonably attractive, eroticized piece of undulating flesh to serve our private purposes.

It had been months since we had worked at even the appearance of a civil relationship, let alone attempted to have sex without cocaine. When our brains were straight we could barely pretend that we even liked each other; only on coke were we "in love."

She hated me for what she perceived as my slothfulness, and I hated her both for her perception and for what I took to be her encouragement of it. She hated me for my friends, particularly my best friend, Michael, whom she hated the most, and I hated her for exploiting them and advancing herself through their reflected glamour. She hated me when I didn't work and when I worked too much, and I hated her for her very presence in my life. Most of all, we each hated the other for a deepening dependency on cocaine — even while we eagerly awaited the other's procurement of a new supply, effusively showered thanks when it was produced, and stole it from each other when it was withheld.

Hatred had become ubiquitous in our lives, yet, with cocaine, we could rid ourselves of it. As the drug purged our brains of our haunting self-doubts and replaced them with a euphoric sense of personal power, it became unnecessary to hate anybody. During the darkest nights of our increasingly poisonous relationship, a few snorts of cocaine could launch us into hours of empathy and deep conversation, even though we had not spoken a civil word to each other for days. Most astonishingly, during these benign hiatuses, we even talked seriously about things like marriage and children. We both knew who we were, we had unlimited confidence, the world lay before us for the taking — so, why not? With the sober mornings that followed those fanciful nights, the answer to the "why not" always became crystal clear.

It was the same with sex. Coke had become essential to both my desire and my performance. Why that should have been so, I don't know for sure; but I have some thoughts about it. There were the erotic fantasies and enhanced tactility that the drug, particularly when taken in combination with others, produced; but there was more to it than that. For a long time — well before Barbara — I had found that my interest in sex was closely related to how I was doing in life generally and how I felt about myself. When things were going well, when I was satisfied with my work, when I felt functional and in control of my life — at those times, my sexual appetite was hardy and its satisfaction rewarding. When problems mounted, when failures occurred and insecurities festered in the unconscious — at those times, the feelings of impotence in life were mirrored, if not by actual impotence in bed, at least by an impotence of the will even to get as far as bed. To be sure, these periods of lassitude often could be "cured" by liquor and maybe a little pot to pacify the anxieties and pique the senses; but, even then, the coupling would be more a routine than an adventure.

Cocaine made me want to screw again. And to undertake any other endeavors requiring an equivalent order of courage. That first morning of the new year of 1979, I felt the rush of power, spun the mobilizing erotic fantasies, and copulated heroically.

Barbara and I lay quietly for a few minutes on the floor, bathed in sweat, exhausted. At about nine in the morning we shuffled our wasted bodies to bed, where in a room made black by shades drawn to reject the sunlight, I spent the "night" as I often did after a cocaine orgy — tossing, turning, and grinding my teeth. It was the time of the drug's aftermath. The glow had dissipated, and all that was left were the seemingly endless hours of nervous tension from a brain still hot wired and implacably at war with a body crumpled by fatigue and desperate for a sleep that refused to come. It was the time when the anxious thoughts returned. *Why* had I spent all that money, and for what? *Why* did I have this woman in bed beside me? *Why* did I pretend to sexual heroism when I knew that true heroism — in bed or anyplace else — was not the forte of a spiritual eunuch? *Why? Why? Why?* It was clear that the party was over. Until the next time.

For the next two days, Barbara and I periodically stumbled out of bed — to get a glass of water or a beer, to go to the bathroom, to swallow without tasting a boiled egg or a piece of dry bread, occasionally to douse our faces with cold water. But finally the recuperation was complete. Early on the third morning of the new year, we got out of bed, showered, and faced the crusted dishes and rotten shellfish that lay stinking in the house from three days past. I asked Barbara why she hadn't cleaned up the mess after our guests had left. She asked me why I hadn't. A fair question. In rejoinder, I said, "Fuck you." She answered in the same vein. We cleaned up without speaking further, and when the unhappy chore was done she stomped wordlessly out the door to her waiting computer. Life was back to normal.

I treated myself to a morning hit. Barbara was gone, so I could enjoy it freely without facing the unpleasant alternatives of either sneaking it or having to give her some. I slid the glass wall open and walked onto the deck. I breathed deeply of the bay's clean air and surveyed the scene. The sky was a Mediterranean blue, the sun was gentle and gave a soft shine to San Francisco's skyline to the south, and the bay lay below like a placid mountain lake without a ripple. I felt refreshed. The demons of doubt had passed. True, there were some minor problems to be dealt with. Barbara, for one. And, my God, the cost of New Year's Eve. With the cocaine, it had run over four thousand dollars. Despite my renewed fortunes, I couldn't pay the rent or the telephone bill. But, no matter, the investment had been worth it. And I would come up with a good way out of any temporary difficulties. I always had. Of late, I had been in a lot worse trouble than this and God had always smiled on me. Now would be no different. I had some solid clients who thought me a miracle worker, and the billings would be big this year. There was no need to fear the precipice; I had been there before, faced disaster down, and come out of the encounters invigorated for new adventure. As for the immediate problems, there was an easy solution. I would bill each of my clients for just a little bit of work that had not quite been completed. They would be none the wiser for that, and ultimately I would give them full value. I took a couple of more hits and felt fine. Yes, there was no question about it. Nineteen seventy-nine was going to be a very good year.

June was unseasonably warm for San Francisco. Despite my inability to shake financial pressures that had become chronic, I had been able to keep my head above water, my cash flow was healthy, my social life was full, and my mood was like the weather — balmy. I still had a number of problems to get rid of, the principal one being Barbara. But that too would pass.

Although it had been four months since we had come to the clear decision to split, we were still together in form if not in substance. The relationship had become more civil because, despite Barbara's lack of will actually to walk away and my benign acceptance of her delays, our feelings and intentions had at least been clarified. I felt a great load lifted from my shoulders; all that remained now was to *act* on the intention.

I had come up with a plan that would both facilitate the break and feed a longtime craving. I would go abroad for a few weeks — ten days or so in France and another ten days in Egypt. I hadn't been to Europe since my army days in the midfifties, and I had never been to the Mideast, and I was full of anticipation at the prospect. Sadat was doing some dramatic things and was emerging as a man of history, great events were in the making, and it would be a journey of learning and excitement. But the trip's *raison d'être* really was the French segment; it would be a time of glamour, romance, elegant wining and dining — in short, the most logical possible extension of my renewed life of privilege.

The precipitating force in all of this — as was usually the case in our group's adventures — was Michael, whose ingenuity in the invention of high-fashion recreation seemed limitless. He was closing a deal for his company in Paris, and it was to be financed with Japanese money. Now, most ordinary mortals would assume that the logical place for such a closing was Chicago. That was where the trustee bank was, where the escrowed money was, and where all the principals could fly in much less time than to France. And the closing, after all, was to be in U.S. dollars, not

French francs. When I pointed all this out to Michael, he replied with the familiar twinkling eyes and very slight smile that signaled the engineering of a coup, "Richard, there are some things you never will understand. This *is* an international transaction, you know, so I'm going to do it *internationally*. I've insisted that these people close the deal in Paris, and that's where they are going to do it." And so they would.

But that would not be the end of it, or — as it turned out — even the beginning. It just happened that the Le Mans twenty-four-hour race was to be a few days before the date for which Michael scheduled the Paris closing. He was going over early to watch his lawyer friend drive in the race, and if *his* friends were really *good* friends, they would go too. After the race we would all go to Paris for a few days of revelry. The night of the closing, we would go to dinner at Maxim's — where we would join the financiers for a dinner that Michael had arranged, but which the bank and the Japanese would pay for. While at Le Mans I would have no expenses since he had rented a large château for himself and his friends.

Michael had been fascinated by car racing for a decade. Those were the years when, if you were upwardly mobile and wanted to make a statement about it, you took up tennis seriously; if you had unequivocally made it, and also wanted it known that you had guts, automobile racing was the thing. Even at fifty, he thought about taking up the sport himself — if not as a driver, then at least as an investor, putting part of his millions into car development and sponsorship. For him, going to Le Mans was a very big deal. And he wanted his friends to share it with him.

So the trip would be a pilgrimage of old buddies sworn to the duties of comradeship. It was an invitation I could not possibly refuse. My life was still burdened with the heavy load of debts that were the aftermath of my Tahoe fiasco, debts that — despite my renewed income — had continued to mount from a series of extravagances needed to feed the appetite of my "success." It was clear that, in the long run, not only my enjoyment of life, but the interests of my creditors as well, could best be served by my continuing to embellish the decorations of a rising status. Cars, clothes, designer furniture, Hawaiian trips, and lavish entertainments were the necessary price of a proper presentation. And, since presentation was everything in business, what folks of a middle-class bent might take as financial improvidence run wild could — when cast in a more sophisticated light — be viewed as the necessary costs of doing business.

There are purchases waiting to be made; the debts will be taken care of when the time is right; everything *will* work out: thus went my daily financial modus operandi. Just recently another new client — the Delaware River Port Authority in Philadelphia — had come to me for my genius in extracting large sums of money from Washington bureaucrats. They needed thirty to forty million dollars to replace the deck on one of their bridges, I clearly was the man for the job, and they would pay well for it. Even more money than I had expected would be coming in. I had already extracted a ten-thousand-dollar payment from the agency on signing the contract. True, it had been spent within a week, but more would come. Yes, I could afford the French adventure — and the additional cost for Egypt would be negligible.

But what about my *true* financial picture? Could I *really* justify the cost of the trip when it would mean another month of delinquent rent, a pile of bills still unpaid, and more borrowed money? These nagging questions did require some serious thinking, so I sat down, had several large snorts, and thought for at least three full minutes.

The answers were clear and reassuring. The trip was mandatory. In fact, there was no way I could afford *not* to go. My obligation of loyalty to Michael would be served — in itself a totally compelling rationalization. But beyond that, there would be many side benefits. I would get away from Barbara, and when I returned she surely would be gone — a smart strategic ploy; I needed the change and I would return refreshed for the serious work ahead; I would have a self-improving cultural experience of great value; and, most importantly, I would be where the action of the moment was — an absolute necessity. It had become clear to me that, above all else, my success, or at least the appearance of it, required being with the action. If I were absent, people might wonder why, and maybe even whisper that I couldn't afford it. And that would never do.

I announced my decision to Barbara, and she said, "That's an absolutely wonderful idea. It will do you a world of good. And it will give us some time apart to get some perspective, and maybe when you get back we'll both feel differently about things." I said, "Yes, and it will give you a chance to look around for a nice place and move without a lot of pressure and anxiety between us."

I had enough money to buy my round trip, first class airplane ticket. After that, I went into a hotel restroom to snort some cocaine. I wanted to jack up my brilliance and confidence before telling my banker that I wanted some more money. It was a small San Francisco bank that I had been doing business with for ten years. The officers were what we referred to as "swinging bankers." That meant that — if you were the right kind of guy — they didn't test you by the standards of credit-worthiness used by the big, conservative banks where stuffiness (which some might call prudence) prevailed. You were the "right kind of guy" if you traveled with the right crowd, had a touch of glamour to your life-style, and made interest payments on your loan often enough — with maybe an *occasional* reduction in principal — to keep the bank examiners off your loan officer's back. That, with occasional drinks and dinner for your loan officer at the fashionable Italian restaurant down the street.

Despite my debt load, I had always taken care of the bank — delinquently, but soon enough to keep myself in their good graces. An occasional interest payment here, a tiny payment on principal there, a funny story and a couple of martinis, and everybody was happy. A month or so later, if necessary, there would always be a few thousand more dollars available to tide me over a "tight period." In this way, my unsecured credit had grown to about twenty thousand dollars, a small amount to some, but a little unusual in my situation, since I was already effectively insolvent and flirting with worse. But, as I drove to the bank, I knew that my needs would be met, and if there were self-doubts, the coke took care of them.

I briefly explained my need for eighty-five hundred dollars for sixty days for some foreign business travel, signed some blank forms (the loan officer could fill them in later), got a cashier's check, deposited it in my account, purchased some traveler's checks, and went shopping. I figured that the eighty-five hundred dollars would do me nicely, since I already had my ticket. Michael was paying for virtually everything in France, and Egypt couldn't cost very much. My American Express card had been revoked, but I still had my MasterCard and Visa, which were becoming very big in Europe. There would be plenty of cash for my needs abroad, and I could afford some preliminary shopping for travel accessories.

The first stop would be at Wilkes Bashford's. A week earlier, at a cocaine party at Mel's, I had had a long talk with a gay hairdresser, who was also his cocaine dealer, about what clothes were hot in France. He had just returned from there and his good taste could be counted on. "Well," Vincent said, "if you're interested in the ladies, as I assume you unfortunately are, the best things to have would be some silk sport shirts, some designer jeans, and a very good pair of cowboy boots. Cowboy boots are very big with the French girls right now." I thanked Vincent for his counsel, offered him some coke from the gram he had just sold me for a hundred and ten dollars, and nervously watched him snort up about a third of it. He thanked me with a winning smile. As instructed, I dropped by the elegant boutique and one of Wilkes's fastidiously beautiful men poured me a glass of wine and we browsed together. In half an hour the casual segment of my travel wardrobe was complete. Five silk sport shirts, four pairs of designer jeans, four Ralph Lauren polo shirts (which, in Wilkes's independent judgment, were obligatory), and a pair of extraordinary hand-tooled cowboy boots — made in Italy.

The second stop was at Greg's house to pick up a good supply of cocaine. I had made a mental list of all the things that had to be done before departure — find my passport, get airplane tickets, get the banking done, shop, get clothes into the cleaners and back on one-day service, get a haircut, pack. But, even with all these tasks to think about, and as I had gone about their accomplishment, one preoccupation transcended all of them. As I drove from the city back to Sausalito, my mind was now able to focus on the transcending issue. How much coke should I buy?

As I drove west on Marina Boulevard, past the long row of Mediterranean-style mansions and the dozens of sailboats moored in the marina, my mind ran through some simple calculations. At Wilkes's prices I had spent a fortune for clothes. That left me with seventy-two hundred. How much coke could I afford and still have a safe amount of cash on location? But the amount I could afford was only one question. The larger one was, How much would I *need?* By now it had become plain that the answers to these two recurring questions in my life were never the same, and — as always — the rules of simple logic selected the obviously right one. The lesser question of affordability must defer to the larger one of need.

Somewhere around the middle of the Golden Gate Bridge, I concluded that an ounce would be about right. That was a lot, particularly since, when the time came, I might be afraid to take the stuff into Egypt, in which case it would all have to be consumed in France. But that wouldn't be hard. I would be frolicking at parties late every night, drinking a good deal, and in need of a lot of energizing. Then there was the race itself — which meant no sleep at all for a twenty-four-hour period. And the Paris entertainments no doubt would be all-night affairs. An ounce — twenty-five hundred dollars' worth in those days — would give me plenty for my own needs, the ability to make some gestures of generosity toward my friends, and still be sure that there was enough of a cushion.

Turning off the freeway onto the Sausalito entry road, I was elated with the heady prospects of the adventures ahead. As I came to the first bend of the curly road that rapidly descended into the bay-level village, I accelerated into it with the élan of a Grand Prix driver, weaving the Porsche with a deft and spirited touch through each successive curve. I flew down a short straightaway, fearlessly added a little shot of power over the hump in the road that caused a dozen wrecks a year, and shot down the remaining hundred yards of the hill. At the bottom I turned left, then another left into Greg's driveway. My new dope dealer, only five minutes from my own house, was a great convenience.

4

Fresh Love and Large Hopes

THE Boeing 747 rose steeply, banked to the west, and headed northeasterly toward the subpolar route that we would follow to London, where I would get an Air France airbus to the City of Light. Altogether, it would be a nine-hour trip, but I didn't mind. Ever since I had graduated from law school, I had spent much of my life on airplanes, flying from my various homes to business-trip destinations that almost invariably were on the opposite coast. Unlike many longtime business travelers, I still loved to fly — even after twenty years of it. And it always felt the same: to be airborne was to be released. As the ground fell away, so did my troubles. Sometimes it was a marriage that wasn't working, sometimes work sitting delinquently undone on the desk, almost always — even in my earlier, more responsible bourgeois years — a stack of bills unpaid. In the air they were all left behind for a while. And always, as the airplane rose higher into the sky, my confidence and feeling of well-being rose with it. Particularly when flying first class.

The No Smoking sign went off and I lit a Salem. It was twilight and the sunset beyond the ocean filled a third of the western sky with a wall of vivid orange. I saw the lights of San Francisco and the city's bridges, sparkling with strings of diamonds, gradually fade away into another part of my past.

A tingling sensation coursed across my cranium, down my neck, and through my body to my toes. It was more than the rush of excitement that comes with the anticipation of new adventures. It was premonition. Of what, I had no idea. If anything singular awaited me, it was not about to reveal its face. But my sense of a decisive turning point ahead was overwhelming.

The captain turned off the seat belt light. The stewardess brought me a double Beefeater martini and took my dinner order. I took a healthy drink, excused myself as I slid in front of my seatmate into the aisle, and went to the restroom. I wiped the aluminum sink counter clean with a paper towel, tapped a mound of powder from my vial onto the counter, cut it into four long lines with the edge of a matchbook, and inhaled the powder — two lines up each nostril — through a short straw. I felt great. Of late, my new dealer, Greg, had been selling mediocre coke. (You could always divine his financial condition from the quality of coke he sold you: when he was on the shorts, he put an extra diluting cut in it; when he was flush, his coke was good.) But this stuff was fantastic. I peered into the mirror and saw that the eyes didn't look too good. It had been a long, busy day with a lot of snorting, drinking, and smoking. One of the stewardesses, a busty brunette with long legs, vibrated possibilities, so I thought it prudent to fix the eyes with a couple of shots of Visine. That done, I popped a Valium and returned to my seat.

Dinner passed quickly in conversation with my seatmate. "Are you headed for London or are you going on from there?" I asked.

"Going on to Paris — to the air show."

"Oh really; they have a big air show there, do they?"

"Oh God, yes. It's the most important air show in the world. Absolutely fantastic."

"Well, I've been to a couple of air shows myself. Local stuff, but exciting. I had no idea that people traveled halfway around the world to go to one."

He chuckled. "Well, you do if you're in the business. It isn't just for entertainment. There's a lot of that, but business is the thing."

"Oh, you're in the airplane business," I said. "You a pilot, designer, or what?"

"Well, I used to fly a lot, but now they've got me parked behind a desk. Air Force."

I looked at the man more closely. Fiftyish, graying hair, tanned, and neatly packaged in Brooks Brothers summer worsteds. Crisp in conversation but friendly. No need to impress; he knew who he was.

"Excuse me, gentlemen," the stewardess said. "Would you like another drink? Mr. Smart?"

"Pardon me? Oh yes — another martini, please."

"And for you, General?"

"Nothing more right now, thank you."

Christ! Wouldn't you know it. Here I am with a couple of grams of coke in my pocket and over two thousand dollars' worth of the stuff in my carry-on bag, and the airline's got me seated next to a goddamn general of the United States Air Force. Well, so what — that's not the same as a cop. No? Maybe not, but they're all on the same side. Oh come off it; what's there to worry about? Recline your seat and enjoy. Bullshit! If this guy has even the hint of a suspicion — what with me running to the bathroom every fifteen minutes and coming back with powder on my nose — he'll turn me in to the pilot in a second. I'll get busted the minute I walk off the plane. You're getting paranoid again; this guy doesn't give a damn about you or how many times you go to the bathroom.

"What's taking you to Europe?"

"What — what? Oh, I'm sorry; I guess I was dozing off. What did you say?"

"I'm sorry," he said, "I didn't mean to disturb you. I was just asking you why you are going to Europe."

"Oh, yes. Well, uh, I'm going to Le Mans. You know, the big twenty-four-hour enduro next week. Actually, I'm a lawyer, but, uh, as a hobby — well, actually it's more than that; sort of a semiprofessional avocation that involves some fun and a few tax write-offs, if you know what I mean — I'm involved in car racing."

"No *kidding*," he said with enormously heightened interest, and I knew I was in trouble. "Are you driving?"

"Well, uh, no — not this year. No, not this year. But a couple of my people are. This year, I'm, uh, just contenting myself with some questions of car technology and related business interests, if you know what I mean."

"Oh hell yes," he said, now thoroughly engaged. "You've got me where I can feel it. What kind of cars are you sponsoring? I used to drive myself, and it was one of the greatest times of my life."

"Porsches," I said, hoping that was the end of it.

"What model?" he asked.

"Excuse me," I said. "I have to go to the bathroom."

I stood in the tiny, suddenly suffocating bathroom, bent over with my elbows resting on the sink counter and my face cupped in my hands. Why was I doing this? Why was I doing it *again?* Why couldn't I answer a simple question with a forthright answer? *Why?* Why the attacks of paranoia when I was carrying coke? Followed only minutes later by an elaborate conning of the man whom I had so irrationally feared just because he symbolized responsibility and duty. Why the need to impress? I didn't know him yesterday and I wouldn't know him tomorrow. I had engaged his interest and that was nice, but the next morning he wouldn't care less whether the guy he had met on the plane was a racing mogul or a potato farmer. *Why?* Well, it must just be one of the dilemmas of flying first class. Probably everybody lies in first class.

I doused my face with cold water to get rid of the sweat,

had a couple of huge hits of cocaine, and took another Valium. I felt better. I smiled at the general and explained to him that, for the first couple of days on long journeys, my system gets all screwed up; hence my frequent trips to the bathroom. "I guess that would play hell with a fellow flying a B-52 on a long-range mission," I said. He laughed. "Well," I said, "I'm drained and have to get a little sleep." He nodded appreciatively, and I didn't have to come up with the model number of the racing Porsches. That was good, since I had not an inkling.

Although my eyes stayed closed until we were awakened for the morning arrival in London, it was not a peaceful flight. If you get it just right — if you achieve that perfect balance of cocaine, booze, and tranquilizers — the night can pass in sweet reverie, with the mind poised delicately on the brink of sleep but still vaguely conscious of the awake world and receptive to its gentler stimuli. Done right, it is a time for the conscious spinning of the dreams you *want*, which are far better than those dreams that are thrust upon you from some unknown, and often hostile, black pit of deep and natural sleep. But tonight, I hadn't got it right; there had been far too much coke and booze, and not nearly enough tranquilizer. My overcharged brain churned relentlessly with unwanted voices and images. I had been careless with the formula, and my favorite fantasies ignored my conjurings. In their stead — as increasingly had been the case of late — there came the demons.

The train pulled out of the Montparnasse station headed for Le Mans. It had been a hellish morning, and I struggled to stop the shaking that had started in the taxi from Charles de Gaulle Airport. I wiped the sweat from my clammy forehead with a shirt sleeve and concentrated on breathing deeply. I hadn't had an hour of natural rest in three days. It had taken every ounce of my waning strength to get this far and, now that I had, I didn't want to die in a train compartment in a foreign land, alone and unlamented.

Gradually, my breathing evened out, my trembling stopped, and survival seemed likely. I was gagging occasionally from a low-grade nausea. I felt crushed by fatigue, and a dull headache pushed out from my brain to fill my eyes and sinuses — the familiar consequence of countless lines of cocaine snorted up into my head in two short days that seemed a year. But despite the throbbing, the taste of bile in my throat, and the pervasive dullness of my body, I finally felt calm and newly eager. My body would recover; it always had. And I was in France. At last. Although my exhausted body cried for the relief of sleep, I told it to hold up for just a bit longer. It would be only a little over two hours to Le Mans, and to sleep now on a short train ride on my first day in this land of romance would be an affront both to the country and to the idea of adventure itself. It was time to revive myself. I took my toilet kit from my carry-on bag and headed to the WC compartment. I had consumed all of the coke in my pocket vial while on the plane; now it was necessary to tap into the larger stash that had been concealed for the trip — a task that required some patience.

A week earlier I had discussed with a friend who was also making the trip some of the crucial advance-planning aspects, not the least of which was how best to transport cocaine into Europe without risking a bust going through customs. Every week, the paper reported somebody getting busted carrying drugs in international travel. Only a few days before we were to leave, the *Chronicle* had carried a story about a movie producer caught with a couple of ounces when departing from the Frankfurt airport. He had taped the stuff to his back in a number of plastic bags. The problem was that they kept putting him through the metal detector, and every time they did he rang all the bells. He finally had to strip, and there the stuff was. His

fatal error: He had used metallic tape. So there you were —
a good idea gone awry with a dumb mistake.

I had sought the expert counsel of Greg the drug dealer,
who ridiculed the very asking of the question. "Come on,
Richard, don't be dumb and make a big melodrama out
of taking some coke into France with you," he said. "Just
take it. That's right, take it on your *person*. The way most
of these jerks get caught is by inventing 'secret' hiding
places in their luggage, which take the narcs about thirty
seconds to sniff out. Carry it *on* you; don't even put it in
your hand-carried luggage. Wear a sportcoat and tie, and
stick the stuff in your inside coat pocket. Your entry form
says you're a lawyer, you'll be well-dressed and looking
good. If they look at anything, it'll be your luggage. They
aren't going to search your person. Just look the bastards
straight in the eye, toss them a *bonjour*, and sail right
through. No big deal at all."

I had come to trust Greg in many things, but not this
one. His cheeky system of international cocaine transport — which was no system at all — was typical of his
general philosophy of almost flaunting his trade, right up
to the brink of disaster. Well, that kind of élan was okay
for him; he had long since been living on the fringes of
society, but I was smack in the middle of it. There was
no way I was going to go sauntering through French customs carrying twenty-five hundred dollars' worth of coke
on me, although the idea did make a certain amount of
primal sense. No, there had to be a *plan*.

My friend had independently been consulting with his
own experts, and the answer was Johnson's Baby Powder.
"What you do is get a can of baby powder, pry the top
off with a screwdriver, pour the powder into a glass, roll
your plastic coke bag up very tightly and seal it with Scotch
tape, stick it in the can, and pour the powder back into
the can. The powder will fill in around the sides of the
coke bag and over the top of it. Put the top of the can back

on. If a customs guy shakes the can, he'll get baby powder. If he takes the top off, all he'll see is baby powder. What do you think?"

"It sounds great. But how do I explain the fact that I don't have a baby with me?"

"Richard, don't be dumb," he said. "Adults use baby powder for all kinds of things — to put in their socks, under their arms, in their crotches — all kinds of things."

If there was anybody who wouldn't screw up on so singular a matter, it was my well-traveled, always wired friend. So, now, in the train's WC, I sat intently on the toilet, gradually prying off the top of a can of Johnson's Baby Powder with one of the small, outfolding arms of a pocket nail clipper. It was painstaking work, and while I pried, I thought about the morning's anxieties. An hour before landing in London I had been jerked into full consciousness by the horrible smell of the breakfast that the stewardess had set in front of me. Immediately the fear had hit. *What the hell am I doing with all this coke, anyway? This Johnson's Baby Powder bit is the stupidest damn idea anybody ever had. That's the first place they'll look. Especially since I had to use two cans instead of one to handle the volume. "Excuse me, sir, but this is passing strange. Why does your toilet kit contain only a razor and two cans of baby powder? Where, might we ask, are your deodorant, toothpaste, toothbrush, and toilet water, sir?"*

Tragic as it would be, there was only one thing to do — dump the stuff. Three times within a half-hour I had taken my toilet kit to the WC, intent on throwing the cans into the trash receptacle before we touched down. And three times I had returned to my seat without having done the deed. The sense of danger was overwhelming, and I was almost certain that I would be caught, but I couldn't bring myself to throw away a three-week supply of the best coke I had ever had.

In London, the customs check had turned out to be

perfunctory. At Heathrow, in the midst of the chaos of a baggagemen's strike, the English had simply asked a couple of obligatory questions of each passenger, and passed us through with a jolly word and a wave. Approaching Charles de Gaulle, however, the terror had hit me again with an even greater intensity; and, once inside the airport, I had foreseen certain doom. Numerous grim-looking, short, uniformed men with pencil mustaches and flat-topped hats with brims in front were apparently engaged in official tasks in and around the immigration desks. I had gotten in line, scared to death. One of the men with a pencil mustache had looked solemnly at my passport, handed it to a second, who stamped it, and waved me through.

I had steeled myself for the next row of desks — the customs check area — prepared for the worst. But there wasn't a customs check — only a single unmanned desk with a sign that said something like "Passengers with items to declare." All the passengers were moving out briskly, some apparently to pick up luggage and others directly toward the taxi stand. "Excuse me," I said to a hurrying passenger, "where is the customs check?" "Oh," she said, "they hardly ever do it here anymore," and ran off. I stood there for a moment, stunned, and felt I was going to faint. The fear and paranoia had been for nothing. Unknowingly, I had been the beneficiary of what I would come to learn was an old French tradition: for every four bureaucrats standing around in uniforms looking officious, only one would actually be doing something.

I had the top of the can off now and, shaking the baby powder into the toilet, I smiled at my recollection of the morning's silly fears. It was still there, my carefully rolled and sealed plastic bag with its load of energy and euphoria. I took the bag out of the can, brushed off the residual baby powder with some toilet paper, unrolled the bag, dipped my house key into it, and snorted my relief from the tip of the key. I resealed the bag, stuck it into my

127

sportcoat pocket, and tossed a couple of codeine pills far back into my throat without benefit of water. I sat a few minutes on the toilet, smoking a cigarette and waiting for the magic. By the time the cigarette was finished, the headache was gone and — although my fatigue was too deep for even coke to dispel entirely — I felt wonderfully well again.

As I walked back to the compartment, haggard, unwashed, unshaven, and rancid mouthed — but nonetheless clad in my silk shirt, designer jeans, Bill Blass sport jacket, and hand-tooled Italian cowboy boots — it felt good to be part of the privileged elite. I had completely forgotten that, but a few hours earlier, I had been perfectly prepared to risk years in prison for the continued comfort of my indispensable traveling companion in the little plastic bag. During those hours, my attitudes and behavior had been precisely those of a common — and very incompetent — criminal.

It was the early evening of my fourth day in France that some friends and I found ourselves in our rented Peugeot, speeding along Anjou's delightful, impossibly narrow farm roads to a place called Château de Teildras, where Michael was hosting a pre-race dinner. Our hearts were light and we were as gay as schoolchildren escaped from classes for a picnic in the country. My San Francisco lawyer friend, James, had at last begun to resolve the constipation he invariably suffered in his first days of culture shock in all foreign places, and with his relief his spirits had soared. And his wife, Catherine, was simply in heaven. A cultivated woman of many enthusiasms and the only linguist in the entire entourage, she had spent her days in unceasing, animated, and often hysterical chatter with each and every Frenchman she could find — peasants, road workmen, shopkeepers, cheese merchants — anybody. Her wide-eyed and unrestrained engagement with the people and the place had been contagious, and, with the surrender of my studied sophistication, I felt like a boy on his first adventure away from home.

It was supposed to be only a seventy-five-kilometer drive, but after an hour and a half, we began to reap only frustration. Maps of French provinces are mind-boggling crazy quilts of meandering roads, right angles that appear to go everywhere and nowhere, apparently purposeless intersections, and randomly scattered dots of villages, whose sheer number suggests that every French family residing in the same locale for three generations has qualified for its very own town. There is no road or cluster of buildings too inconsequential to escape the notice of a French mapmaker.

Were it not for the soft beauty of the farms, painted with the fading gold light and lengthening shadows of early evening, we might well have abandoned the nerve-fraying search in favor of a bracing cognac in some forlorn country bar. But that, too, would have been impossible; deep in French farm country apparently everything closes up tight by six. Every gray village we passed through was dark, every shutter closed; the streets were emptied of life. As our trip became an interminable series of screeching stops, false starts, and wrong turns, we sank into brooding and muttered curses. A quick toot of coke would have picked up my spirits, but James and Catherine were not among the initiates. There was nothing I could do to relieve the growing fatigue and frustration without risking an unpleasant scene.

Michael's instructions had told us to look for a village called Cheffes-sur-Sarthe, and suddenly, with all our pointless meanderings and strained patience, there it was, indistinguishable from all the other gray villages we had passed through. We slowed to look for the sign to the château and found it. James turned the car to the north. Immediately on our right there loomed an ancient and ugly cemetery crammed to overflowing with tilted, de-caying monuments. The decrepit cemetery, with its time-blackened angels and corroded crucifixes, some horribly askew above the bones they guarded, seemed an awful shadow image of the town, where the inhabitants were surely living people but which, to all appearances, was dead itself. Objectively, the scene may not have been that terrible, but it had been five or six hours since I had had any cocaine. I was suddenly into one of the worst depres-sions I had ever experienced, overwhelmed by my des-perate need for a snort. I had come to France for life, not death.

We crossed a cement bridge over a small stream, as Michael's directions had said we would, and knew that we were almost there. Almost immediately past the bridge, the bumpy road became a lovely avenue bordered by hedges and trees whose branches arched over us. Ahead of us, through the trees on our left, Teildras rose with simple dignity from a small plateau at the far side of a lush meadow ringed with ancient great oaks. Above the sloping slate roof with its oval stone window dormers, several chim-neys, and modest towers, a long, gentle hill lush with the green leaves of June leaned into a soft sky that was still alive with the rich blue of early evening.

On the slightly raised plateau beyond the meadow, I glimpsed perhaps a dozen people seated, presumably with drinks, at round tables that supported huge beige um-brellas that looked like butterfly wings against the sky. Separating the meadow from the courtyard of the château was a low stone wall where rosebushes and plants blos-somed in a symphony of color. If by sorcery the scene could instantaneously have been transferred to canvas, the Louvre would have taken it without question as a genuine Degas, except of course for the anachronism of the ladies' and gentlemen's attire. I felt a tinge of delight. The cloud of depression that had gathered only minutes earlier had lifted, and suddenly the world looked fresh.

The driveway took us into a finely graveled parking area at the front of the great house. We entered by way of a sitting room, where we were enveloped by history and greeted by the host. Probably about seventy years old, he was well over six feet tall, and had the look of a man who, despite his age, had a hard, muscular body beneath his baggy but casually elegant clothes. His face, with its high forehead and long Roman nose, said, "There are no frills or embellishments in this person; what you see is what you get." Dressed in gray flannel slacks, tweed sportcoat, tattersall shirt, plain wool tie, and cashmere sweater, he was a distillation of both understated charm and absolute control. A proud aristocrat forced by circumstances to convert his beloved family house into a country inn, he was not, his manner clearly indicated, a man of commerce, but a gentleman of unassailable dignity having a few friends in for dinner.

"Good evening, madame *et* messieurs. Please come in; it's nice to have you with us. Some of your friends are already here. If you like, we can go outside — it's a lovely evening — and have a cocktail." He spoke a serviceable and beautifully accented English.

I very much wanted a drink and was anxious to join the rest of the party, whose bright laughter from the courtyard promised a happy time. But more than anything else, at the moment I wanted — no, *needed* — some cocaine.

"*Ah, monsieur, où sont les toilettes, s'il vous plaît?*"

A fleeting, kindly smile. "You'll find the bathroom down at the end of that hall and to your left," he said in English. Well, I thought, I had tried, and the old gentleman looked as though he appreciated the effort.

I made sure the door was locked and took the film canister from my pocket. Over the last half-hour or so, I had become increasingly agitated, and my hand was shaking as I pried off the rubber top. I made four huge lines on the marble slab that the two sinks were set into, snorted them deeply into my nostrils as quickly as possible, and took a Valium. I leaned against a wall, rolled my head far back on my shoulders, and while I looked at the ceiling breathed deeply and slowly. In a couple of minutes I felt fantastic. But despite the quick shot of euphoria and the glow of well-being that seemed to suffuse every cell of my body, an anxiety was gnawing away somewhere inside. That wasn't supposed to happen; the coke was supposed to dispel all negative intrusions. What wasn't working?

I had been doing so well the past three days — a fair amount of sleep, good food, a lot of exercise, and, most significantly, very little cocaine. Why now, after feeling so healthy and in control of my body, this almost hysterical compulsion to get to the coke, even before saying hello to my friends outside? And what about those few seconds of black despair, even fear, as we motored into the bleak village of Cheffes and passed the cemetery? The reaction had been wholly out of proportion to the reality. Had I an intimation of psychosis? Had it anything to do with the drug? Nonsense, I decided, all nonsense. A weird but short aberration of the mind in a strange place, and it had passed as quickly as it had come. With my first view of Teildras and the scene of bucolic richness, my spirit had soared; everything had quickly come right. And yet, there remained the fact that, with the prospect of a perfect night before me, I *had* had that irresistible compulsion — with an intensity I had never before experienced — to get myself heavily stoked up before talking to *anybody* or enjoying *anything*.

Forget it. My mind was playing dumb tricks with dark mirrors. It was time to knock off the morbid self-analysis and get on to the festivities. I was using the coke only to make good things better, and that was all there was to it.

132

I was sure of that because by now the cocaine and Valium had settled in nicely, and had brought reason to my internal dialogue. Everything was fine. In fact, it was positively great. For the first time I took note of the bathroom ambience — finely shaded marble sink, elegant wallpaper, burnished gold faucets, delicately molded pastel soaps, and a selection of fine toilet waters. I patted a little Paco Rabanne on my beard and neck, took another couple of hits of cocaine, glowed, smiled, and thought, "Oh yes, this is going to be a fine time."

Michael had happened onto Teildras quite by accident a week earlier. Discovering upon his arrival that the "château" the travel agent had rented him was in fact a huge, ramshackle farmhouse, he had immediately set out to find more suitable accommodations. He hadn't been able to get a room at Teildras, but, taken with the charm of the place, he had booked the dinner and reported to me, with great earnestness, that "not only is the place fantastic, it also has *daughters*. Beautiful daughters. *French* daughters. Charming, flirtatious, and, for all I could tell, unattached. "Richard," he said, "you simply have got to make a move for one of those daughters. The Maxim's dinner is going to be a triumph. You simply cannot be alone in Paris. This is your chance. *Get one of those Dubois sisters.*"

I had nodded tolerantly without taking it very seriously. Everybody wanted me to be in love — or at least a reasonable facsimile thereof and for however short a time. And I wasn't averse to the idea myself. But seduction was easier said than done, even in France — maybe *especially* in France. I wasn't counting on it. At any rate, the question of the Dubois sisters and what Richard was going to do about them had become a cause célèbre among our group, both a running joke and a matter of some serious interest. (As it happened, these mysterious delights were not the "Dubois" sisters at all — a piece of information that subsequently would cause me no little embarrassment. Dubois

133

apparently was the only French name Michael could keep in his mind or pronounce.)

So I sat with friends in gracefully turned natural wood armchairs set around wood tables under widely spread beige parasols, breathing the cool evening air, basking in the twilight, and gazing out across an expansive green meadow textured with the lengthening black shadows of great oaks planted three or four centuries ago. And everywhere, flowers. I sat waiting for a drink and the appearance of one or the other of the renowned "Dubois" sisters. As it happened, I would not have long to wait for either.

She was very blond, her hair hanging straight to the shoulders, with Dutch-cut bangs across the forehead. High cheekbones, forthright eyes, and a gently tapering chin. A wide, sensuous, and beautifully proportioned mouth. From the nose, large but handsome, it was evident that she was indeed the father's daughter. Except for her small stature, she looked more Scandinavian than French. But when she spoke, in nicely accented English, there was no doubt of her Frenchness. "Please, monsieur, would you care for a drink?"

"Yes, thank you, a dry martini I think. On ice, please."

"Of course," she said, looking a little puzzled.

I watched her walk back to the house. She was wearing a simple emerald green shift that hung straight from her shoulders and the lift of her breasts. It was a no-nonsense dress designed for work rather than enticement or play. The quality of the body could only be guessed at, but the slender, long-muscled arms and the smallness of the ankles suggested that the undisclosed was a risk well worth taking. The other sister was nowhere about — out of town, I later learned — but her absence was of no consequence; this one would do nicely. The problem was how to approach her. She was handsome and charming and remote.

An opening for some bright repartee came moments later when she returned with a long-stemmed glass full of a sticky red liquid with a tiny, forlorn cube of ice in it. I took it, sipped it, grimaced in a definite but, I thought, inoffensive way, and said, "My dear, I do not know what this is, but it definitely is not a martini, and it really is quite terrible. Here, you see, is how we make a dry martini on ice. We take a pre-chilled glass and put three or four fresh ice cubes in it. We then fill the glass with pre-chilled gin, and to that we add just a drop of dry vermouth. When that is done, we put either a small piece of lemon peel or a green olive in the glass — if a lemon peel, we gently rub it around the rim of the glass first. *That* is a martini."

I had meant it to be amusing. The girl in the green dress was not amused. "You asked for a martini," she said. "I personally poured it out of a Martini bottle. *That* is a martini."

I chuckled lightly and made a great show of patience. "Ah, now I understand the confusion," I said. "What we have here is a glass full of sweet vermouth poured from a bottle labeled Martini and Rossi, which is why *you* thought you were making a martini. No, a martini is made of gin with just a *touch* of vermouth. *Dry* vermouth."

Her jaw was tightly clenched and her eyes burned. "I'm very sorry, *sir* [the "monsieur" had been conspicuously dropped], I'm not entirely familiar with American drinking habits. We have many people here, and I have to serve some other drinks now; perhaps you would be more comfortable if I just brought you a large bottle of gin and a bucket of ice." She didn't say it; she hissed it. I had lost her. She didn't like me at all. And I never saw my dry martini.

The first great anticipation of the evening was how I would make out with one or the other (maybe both?) of the "Dubois" sisters. The other was the purported coming of Paul Newman. With Rolf somebody-or-other, Germany's premier Porsche driver, Newman was co-driving one of the three cars entered at Le Mans from the same racing stable that had rented a car to Michael's friend. Michael had gotten to know Newman casually around American tracks, and he had cajoled the owner of the cars into producing Newman at the dinner. At least, so he said. Michael was a genius at this sort of thing, and maybe he could do it; but folks weren't holding their breath. Usually Michael pulled off his grandiosities, but occasionally they fizzled. This one, at best, was a fifty-fifty bet. The hour was late, dinner was approaching, and still no Paul Newman. But everybody was hoping. "Paul," Michael had repeatedly said, "is a great guy. You'll enjoy him." Yes, and he also was a dynamite movie star, which didn't hurt. Everybody, behind their studied fronts of blasé indifference, wished mightily that it would come to pass.

And so it did. There he came at last, ambling through the Roman arch into the courtyard, lean, lightly tanned, with his jacket slung over his shoulder just like Hud. No, just like Paul Newman. The women were beside themselves — that's not fair; the men were too. But — except for suddenly lowered voices — everybody was too cool to show it. Just another megastar come to dinner, folks. He walked around the far side of the courtyard looking at the flowers, then into the house, then out again — just kind of wandering around. Nobody went up to say hello because nobody wanted to appear to be a celebrity hound; *that* would be distinctly *un*cool. I finally decided that *that* was nonsense. The poor man was as uncomfortable in his celebrity as all these sophisticated folks were dumbfounded by his presence. All he wanted to do was sit down, have a drink, and talk to real people. Well, *I* would put Paul Newman at ease. But first I would have a couple of toots of coke. It was not that I actually *needed* it just to say hello to Paul Newman. It just was the time, that's all; the glow was starting to wear off, anyway.

I hurried to the bathroom, had a couple of good hits,

and felt just fine. Once again, the drug was reliable, the most loyal of companions. No more of that nervousness that I had felt in the company of high school football heroes when my best shot was on the debate team. No more of the anxiety felt as a twenty-eight-year-old lawyer on Wall Street (did they or did they not think me good enough to become a partner?). Not a shadow of a doubt about my talent, integrity, or worth to the world. With a good dose of high-quality cocaine, I could be sitting at dinner with the pope on my right, David Rockefeller on my left, and the reincarnation of Eva Perón across the table, and I would be right where I belonged.

"Hello," I said with an extended hand. "You look like Paul Newman and walk like Paul Newman, so you must be Paul Newman. I'm Richard Smart." (I had rehearsed it, and it sounded good.)

"That's what *you* say," he said, "but you don't look like Richard Smart, you don't walk like Richard Smart, and I doubt that you really are Richard Smart, but I'll have to take your word for it. Good to meet you." We laughed, I took hold of his elbow and said, "Let's get a drink." Paul Newman had a friend for the night, and I had a status symbol. It was a good deal all around.

It was a night of perfection. There were eighteen of us at three tables — eight at mine, including Paul Newman. Since I had commandeered the celebrity, the more interesting members of the group naturally gravitated to my table, while the others managed to assuage the indignity of their seating with some of the most exquisite food in France. The girl in the green dress took food orders while Le Comte — still every inch the aristocratic host — suggested the wines. It was evident that the family of the house was unused to handling such a group — all sitting for a dinner at once, competing for the attention of the girl in the green dress to get translations of the menu, shouting "More wine please, more wine please," and generally having an uproariously good time. But, with all the chaos, the family and the boisterous guests quickly merged in a festive mood of classless camaraderie in which innkeepers and clients were one.

The family appreciated our naïve enthusiasm for their house, their food, and their attentiveness — a welcome relief, I was to learn, from the supercilious attitudes of the French bourgeoisie, who delighted in an evening of servitude by a family of displaced nobility turned into innkeepers; and a positive *joy* compared to the *English*, toward whom the traditional French — I was astonished to learn — nourish a centuries-old enmity surpassing even that held for the Germans. Agincourt, it seems, sticks in the French craw harder than the incursions of the Bosch. It wasn't that English guests weren't *nice;* they were *too* nice. That and the fact that, no matter how well educated, they refused to speak French; at least the Americans could be excused because they didn't know how. The English waltzed into the château with an air of condescension that suggested that France really belonged to them, if only history could get itself straightened out. And, since the French felt that England was properly *theirs*, it was an emotional stalemate that did not make for happy entertainments. Besides, Le Comte — an old naval officer — had never forgiven Churchill's destruction of the French fleet. "An outrageous act," he said, "taken under the pretense of a need to keep the ships from falling under German control, but actually a malicious English plot to eliminate the French navy as an element of power in postwar politics." But that was a nicety of revisionist history that I was not to learn from Le Comte until some months later.

We ate, drank, talked, and laughed until well past midnight. The wine flowed freely and the food came hot, delicate, and exquisite, although not without some amusing chaos. My plate of thinly sliced duck covered with a dark but lightly textured sauce, and complemented with richly colorful vegetables, looked like a carefully crafted painting. The French have raised not only the preparation, but also the presentation, of food to high art, and the visual beauty of the plate was as affecting as their flower gardens. If my palate got as much pleasure from the food as my eye had, it would be a marvel. I tasted a bite of the duck and it was superb. Unfortunately, it was not duck.

The girl in the green dress was directly across the table from me, serving Newman another beer. "Excuse me, mademoiselle," I said, "this really is delicious — *really* it is; but I think there has been a small mistake."

"Oh?" Eyebrows raised. "What is the problem?"

"Well, you see, I ordered *canard* — that *is* duck, isn't it? As opposed to *poulet*, which, if I recall correctly, is chicken. Do I have that right? Yes? Well, then, the problem is this. I definitely did order duck — *canard*, I mean — and this, I am absolutely certain, is *poulet*. Absolutely delicious," I hastened to emphasize once more, "but chicken nonetheless."

She just stood there for a long minute, looking at me very levelly, with eyebrows raised and lips puckered forward in an expression that indicated a sincere search for a solution. She took a deep breath, leaned clear across the table, balanced herself with her hands resting on either side of my plate, and brought her face level with my own, only a foot away. She looked deeply and seriously into my eyes. "Monsieur," she whispered with one corner of her mouth slightly tightened in an expression of great confidentiality. "I have looked at your plate very carefully and you are right. That definitely is chicken, not duck. I'm sorry, but you see we are just simple country people, we are not used to serving this big a crowd all at once, and it is all very confusing for us. At this very moment, poor Bernard, our simple waiter, is sitting in the kitchen, his head in his hands, almost in tears because he can't get the orders straight. But I'm going to tell you a secret that will make you feel better." Her eyes grew wide as saucers, and she leaned still closer. "*Poulet, canard;* chicken, duck," she whispered, "what does it really matter? In this place *they all taste the same.*"

And there she stayed, with her face thrust over my plate, her eyes wider than ever staring into my own, and her lips sucked in between her teeth — a look that said more eloquently than any words could, "There, Mr. Smart-ass, if it's repartee you want, what have you got to say that's cleverer than *that?*" And I had nothing — nothing at all. Suddenly a great laugh exploded from her pursed lips. She brought herself upright, threw her head back as far as it would go, rolled her eyes, gasped, and brought her hand to her mouth, struggling to contain her hilarity and, at the same time, feigning horror at her mock slander of her mother's cuisine. She quickly moved off, but tossed a glance over her shoulder, smiling, flushed, and shaking with silent laughter. I decided that, having won with great style, she had put the martini incident out of mind and maybe, in fact, even liked me.

It was one in the morning and time to go. It had been a splendid time, most of which I had spent either trying to flirt with the girl in the green dress or talking to Newman. He had proved a delightful dinner partner; there had been talk of politics, disarmament, EST, and the human potential; talk of race cars and sawing Robert Redford's car in half on his birthday; talk of sailboating around the Aegean with his wife, Joanne, and Gore Vidal; talk of wives and children and the fullness of life. But yes, it was time to go. First a trip to the bathroom for one last toot to facilitate the ride back to my lodgings. I took the lid off the canister and looked inside. I couldn't believe what I saw — almost nothing. It wasn't possible. I had loaded the thing in the afternoon with three grams, and all that was left was enough for a tiny whiff. Where had it all gone? Sure, I had made four or five trips to the bathroom during the evening, but I always did that, and never in my life had I used that much cocaine in so short a period. And I didn't *feel* that I was using any more than usual. Well, I was going to have to watch it. No problem.

Walking to the car with James and Catherine, I breathed deeply of the cold night air and looked up at the stars that shimmered in a jet black sky. Somewhere across the meadow a night bird was singing in a round, mellow alto. It had, quite simply, been the finest night of my life, and I was sad to see it end. Most of all, I was depressed at having failed to make a move on the girl in the green dress. It was not that I sensed the tragic loss of a great romance that might have been; only that I craved the joy, however transient, of an authentic small one. Here I was in the country that, according to the storybooks, had civilized the brief encounter and persuaded the world that, when done in France, even a one-night stand exalts the soul. She would have been perfect — full of life, clever, so-phisticated, and (I had concluded from a night of careful study of the movements underneath the baggy green dress) very well put together. Well, it was all fantasy anyway; best to forget about it. This was a very proper family, clearly of the old school, and my chances of persuading her to run off for a time with a horny American who couldn't even speak the language were, as a practical mat-ter, nil. By morning, she'd be forgotten. Out of sight, out of mind.

"C'mon, Richard, let's go compliment the chef."

We were all a little drunk, except James, who was very drunk. Just as we reached the end of the courtyard, James stopped, grabbed my arm, and insisted that we find the kitchen. Catherine and I protested that that wasn't the thing to do, it was very late, the people were tired and glad at last to be rid of us, and, in any event, it was not really sophisticated to go barging, uninvited and unannounced, into somebody else's kitchen, no matter how good the food was.

"Oh, bullshit," James slurred. "This is a great country, these are great people, and it was great food. What you're supposed to do is compliment the chef. Believe me, they'll appreciate it." There was no stopping him, and he dragged me through a doorway that did indeed put us smack in the middle of the kitchen.

She was standing right in front of us. "Hello," James slurred, "I'm James and this is my friend Richard. We had such a great time and enjoyed the evening and the food so much that we just wanted to tell you so."

"Well, thank you, that is very kind. We had a wonderful time too. It was a lot of fun having you. Good-night."

"Go ahead, Richard, *ask* her."

"Ask her *what?*"

"Ask her *out.*"

Oh, my God, I thought, this really is embarrassing. He wasn't even whispering.

"Mademoiselle," I said, "I don't know if you're interested in car racing, but Le Mans is the day after tomorrow and I would very much like it if you'd watch the race with me."

Suddenly there was a fourth person in the conversation. A very small, slender woman I thought to be in her mid-sixties had appeared from nowhere and, vigorously waving her hands about as only the French can do, was speaking with some agitation, and no English, to the girl in the green dress. She was wearing a stark black, elegant dress with an apron over it and an extraordinary white pearl necklace. Her long gray hair was pulled tightly back from a strong, thin face — an effect that accentuated the severity of her expression. I gathered that she was not pleased.

The girl responded with equally rapid French and flying hands, going on forever it seemed to me in my growing nervousness. Finally she patted the older woman on the shoulder, gave her a saucy little smile, and waved the back of her hand at me three or four times as you do when you are shooing a cat away. The elegant old lady shot me a quick glance, muttered, "*Bonsoir, monsieur,*" and moved off to the far side of the huge kitchen where she immediately started shouting orders to the staff, who, as far as I could tell, were quite innocent of any wrongdoing.

"What was all that about?" I asked.

"Oh," she laughed, "that was Mama. She was *very* upset that these strangers are in her kitchen and wanted to know what you are doing here. I told her that you were *so* impressed with her cuisine that you just *had* to express your gratitude. She said that that was nice, but she didn't think that was entirely it. I confessed that, while you really did like her food, you also wanted to take me out. She told me that she suspected as much and told me to act like a lady for a change. I told her that I *am* a lady, that you are very nice, not to worry about it, and that she should go make sure the stale sauces aren't sticking to the pans. And that is what that was all about." She stifled a giggle.

I asked her if her mother always dressed like that when working in the kitchen.

"Of course. Mama is a great lady." I didn't doubt it.

"Well, what do you think about the race?"

"I would love to go. But I have to work at dinner, so I'll have to meet you about midnight."

Going back outside, I was walking on air. I sensed the beginnings of success. The appointed hour of the rendezvous was a bit late by American standards — by normal operating procedures I would have expected to have long since left the track by midnight and be cavorting with the lady beneath a soft down quilt in some remote country inn — but then, when in strange lands, the putative seducer's wise course undoubtedly is to defer to local customs. If she preferred doing it just before breakfast, who was I to protest? I was cold sober now; the thrill of the encounter, and the promise of romance, had cut through the fog of alcohol and cocaine and left me clear-headed and elated.

It was close to three in the morning when we finally pulled into the drive of the decaying farmhouse where we were staying. I washed my face and sat down on the ancient, spineless mattress that, in its terminal illness, groaned and sank to the floor with the first hint of flesh. The old house was quiet as a graveyard. The night's music was gone. There was not even the sound of ice tinkling in glasses, and the air was empty of laughter. The room was badly lit, damp, and cold, and the peeling wallpaper smelled of mildew. I thought of the girl in the green dress and wished she were there. But *nobody* was there. Not my friends, not my wife, not my daughters, not my clients. Where was my father? How old was he now — in his eighties? God, I hadn't talked to him in over a year. It would be good to talk to him; I would have to give him a call when I got back. Everybody — *everybody* — had retreated into the night and I was alone and lonely. It was that time of night again — that dreaded time when the music had stopped and I had only myself. It hadn't always been like that — I hadn't always hated quiet darkness and feared the refuge of sleep. There was no mystery in the change; it had begun with the cocaine. It got you so incredibly high that you simply didn't want to come down.

As coke increasingly had become the regular companion of my waking hours, so had sleep become my endemic enemy. I had come to hate the depth of night, the loneliness, and, most of all, the prospect of bed, for it was in bed that unwelcome thoughts fermented and bubbled most insistently. Just as the drug had magnified the best possibilities of my psyche into images of glittering diamonds, so in its aftermath were my lesser aspects magnified into unsightly lumps of dull black coal. And which, after all, *was* the reality? Who was to say that my sober fears were more real than my cocaine-enlarged hopes? All I knew was that I now *functioned* better on coke than I did without it, and the world functioned with me. And functioning was what life was all about.

The answer was a little more cocaine, which, despite all my aloneness, would quicken my brain again and give me perhaps a glowing hour of revived spirits. I opened my suitcase, removed the plastic bag from the dirty sock that I had hidden it in, and dumped a good-sized pile on the table by the bed. I needed a little wine, too. I knew that, however much I hated the prospect, I needed sleep, and the wine would help it come. Coke to keep me awake and wine to put me to sleep. A confusion? Perhaps. But that's the way it was. I snorted the coke quickly and drank half a litre of the raw country burgundy directly from the bottle. I felt sick, but better. In a few minutes I collapsed on the bed, fully clothed and wasted.

I thought a lot about Paul Newman in the days following our dinner together. A man of talent, sensitivity, and intelligence, he obviously had a deep concern for the important things in life. I had been surprised by his simplicity and genuineness, and captivated by his devotion to his wife. "Joanne" had been at the center of all his conversation. I wondered if I would ever see him again. Originally, and naturally enough, I had been attracted by his celebrity, but my interest had grown beyond that, for here was a celebrity who had his life very much together, a megastar who hadn't been badly affected by fame and fortune, a husband and father who chose to live in Connecticut rather than Malibu. I admired him and envied his creation of a life that wedded glamour and wealth with solid values.

145

The next I heard anything of Paul Newman was almost a year to the day after our dinner together. I was sitting in the same dining room of the same Château de Teildras when I learned that Paul's son, full of drugs, had killed himself. I felt badly for Paul, whom I had known only briefly, and for his dead son, whom I'd known not at all. I thought how awful it was for a young life to have been destroyed by drugs. It was too bad that he wasn't equipped to handle them. I didn't know that, while some such suicides come quickly, others take more time; that some snuff out the life of the body while others slowly corrode the soul.

Although we had, through an embarrassing faux pas, missed connections for Le Mans, I wasn't about to give up on the girl in the green dress. The race was done, but Paris remained — the grand excitement of cathedrals, museums, sidewalk cafés, and, of course, the dinner at Maxim's. A romantic time certainly; but what was romance without a woman? It would be a great thing to pray in Notre Dame, but not half as much fun alone.

So, despite fears of another embarrassment, I sucked up my courage and telephoned the château again. This time Yolaine herself answered, misunderstandings were cleared up, and the gods smiled on me. When I had repeatedly telephoned before the races, her young cousin, who spoke practically no English, had answered and, after the third call, had related to the family the repeated inquiries of a crazy American about some women named Dubois. Yolaine had assumed it was me, had wanted to telephone me back, but had no number. She was not, she explained, a Dubois, but a de Bernard — a de Bernard du Briel, to be exact. I assumed that a proliferation of last names was the mark of something special but, at the time, I was more interested in fashioning the elements of a respectably put, and irresistible, proposition than in the significance of the nomenclature of old French families.

"Mademoiselle, I'm sorry and embarrassed about the confusion."

"Oh, it is no problem," she said. "I had to work quite late and, with the heavy rain, I probably would not have gone anyway."

"However, mademoiselle, there is a lovely event coming up, and I would be most pleased if you would accompany me. I know this may sound very strange, since you hardly know me; but our group is having a large dinner in Paris tomorrow night — at Maxim's — and I think you would enjoy it. Also, I understand you have a lovely sister and . . ."

"What has my sister got to do with it?" she interrupted. There was a sharp bite to the question. Aha, I thought, a hint of jealousy, which must mean interest.

"Oh, only that I have a friend who also is here alone, and I think that your sister would enjoy him." Michael's business associate from Hawaii had arrived the day before the race. He was strikingly handsome, rich, and amusing, and, although the sister had been away during our evening at the château, from what I had heard I was sure they would make a fine couple. "Roy is a very interesting fellow and a gentleman," I said, and then improvised the masterstroke that I was confident would establish me as a considerate man of unquestionable honor. "And, actually, it occurs to me that, considering the circumstances of our only slight acquaintance, you might feel more comfortable coming to Paris in the company of your sister. That was the main reason for my inquiry about her." In truth, I had little doubt that Roy, with his vaunted mastery of the ladies, would have the sister conveniently and blissfully out of the way in no time at all.

There was a moment of silence. "It sounds like a lot of fun. Who will be there?"

147

"Oh, pretty much the same people you met at your home — a really enjoyable group."

Another short silence. "If you'll excuse me for a minute, I'll talk to my sister about it."

"Oh, of course," I said, trying to sound blasé.

There was much rapid French in the background, interspersed with laughter. I could visualize the French hands gesturing nonstop, the shrugs, the raised eyebrows and puckered lips with which these marvelously expressive people adorned their every conversation, no matter how large or small the subject, and while I waited — increasingly confident of the outcome — I smiled at the image of two vivacious young women intensely discussing the pros and cons of a brief fling in Paris, giggling, and plotting their response.

"Is Paul Newman going to be there?"

"*What?*" I said, not even trying to conceal a sudden agitation. I could hardly believe the candid tastelessness of the question, not to mention its implicit insult to my view of myself as the main attraction.

She laughed. "*I'm* not asking," she said. "It's Carole. She's like that."

"Of course," I lied. "Paul wouldn't miss it for the world."

So the arrangements were made.

At seven o'clock, about a dozen of us were sitting in the American Bar of the Ritz Hotel drinking, laughing, having a wonderful time — and awaiting the arrival of the by-now famous "Dubois" sisters. We had come to Paris ahead of them, and the bar was the place for the appointed rendezvous. There had been much unkind skepticism voiced, and a few bets placed, as to whether they would show up. They did.

At the sight of Yolaine, I went a little numb. The baggy green dress had been discarded for silk. The strong face was lightly touched with brushes of shadow and hints of color, yet, through some mystery of arcane feminine art, remained a portrait of natural loveliness. She had a long stride for so small a woman, and, beneath the clinging silk, every line of her legs, hips, and breasts could be followed as they moved with grace, sensuousness, self-assurance, and not a suggestion of vulgarity. In the light of the chandelier, the soft blond hair glistened like a nimbus, and every eye in the bar was on her. She was an astonishing hybrid of innocence and worldliness, of almost unsettling simplicity and high glamour.

She looked at me as levelly as I've ever been looked at in my life, her eyes dancing and seemingly even larger beneath the delicately shadowed lids, and said, "Hello," with a big, ingenuous smile. It was a short greeting but, with its ring of enthusiasm, it was quite enough. I said, "I'm very glad you came," took her hand, and, with subtle aplomb, I thought, lightly brushed my lips across it. "Oh, how very Continental," she laughed.

"Well, we try our best," I said.

It would prove to be a festive night for us, but not so great for Maxim's. Michael's Japanese investors and the Chicago bankers had gone to the restaurant separately, so it was just us Californians and our two French ladies who assaulted the venerable establishment in a blithe and bois-terous mood. We had barely trooped through the door when I sensed something was amiss. The maître d's smile froze on his face, and several of the staff took to whispering and gesticulating in a corner. It was not a glad-handed welcome. The tip-off came — although it was an enigma at the time — when the frosty maître d' hissed, "Well, monsieur, I do hope you and your friends have had a pleasant day hunting in the country." A strange comment, probably an institutionalized code phrase, I thought.

Within a moment of being seated we saw the gentle-man's meaning all too clearly. Seated in the choicest, most visible spot in the entire restaurant, in the center room adjacent to the dance floor, we Californians were surrounded by a room full of elegantly gowned women and men dressed up in very black suits, very white shirts and — among the few who weren't black tie — muted cravats. Our women measured up well; as for Michael, James, and myself, it was simply a disaster. We had thought we were quite natty, with our blazers, tweed sportcoats, and seersucker jackets, nicely set off by striped or checkered shirts and an assortment of happy ties. Unfortunately, nattiness was not Maxim's thing. Michael was humiliated, the other patrons were astounded, Maxim's was mightily pissed, and Yolaine was practically rolling off her chair with laughter.

"Oh, this is wonderful, absolutely wonderful," she kept repeating, while tears of hilarity rolled down her cheeks and streaked her makeup. "I tried to tell you, I really did try." And so she had. At the Ritz bar, when Michael had announced that we should get moving on to dinner, Yolaine had casually asked me if the ladies should wait in the bar while the gentlemen dressed. "Oh, no," I had said, "we're ready to go." "Oh," she had said.

I could feel a hundred pairs of Parisian eyes burning with disapproval. I rested my elbows on the table and buried my face in cupped hands. Yolaine shook me by the arm. "Oh, come on," she said, "this is no major catastrophe. In fact it is absolutely hilarious. Maxim's is the most pretentious, stuffiest restaurant in Paris, if not in the world, and the people who run it are pompous asses. They've never had to deal with anything like this in their lives. They're absolutely paralyzed. They don't know what to do. It's wonderful!" I looked at her with unconcealed awe. Here I was, my carefully polished façade of sophistication collapsed in a heap of tackiness, my hopes of romance crumbled with it, and this beautiful, wonderful girl — in one of those delightful exercises of inverted snobbery that is possible only for those precious few people whose nat-

ural class and grace have made all the world their do-
main — had turned the disaster upside down.

"What I don't understand is how we got in at all with
you and your friends dressed like this." An apologetic
giggle. "And this seating — unbelievable." She took both
my hands in hers, brought her eyes level with mine, and,
as though gently instructing a schoolboy, said, "Now I'm
going to tell you about Maxim's. It's the most expensive
restaurant in Paris, which is its main credential. The food
used to be fantastic; now, it's only passable. But famous
people and Arabs and very rich people — nouveau riche
people mainly and people who pretend to be rich — still
come here because it's *the* place for these kinds of people
to be, simply to congratulate themselves on being here.
Do you understand? Good. And it's a good place to practice arrogance. Besides all that, the place really *is* a lot of
fun, despite the bullshit." The thoughtful description didn't
surprise me, but the easy obscenity did. Yet, coming from
her, even *bullshit* sounded musical — especially since it
came out *boolsheet*.

"But the thing is, hardly anybody *ever* comes in here
for dinner without a dark suit, and *never* — not *ever* — on
a Friday night, when black tie is really the thing. They
simply won't let you in. But even if you're *dressed* for
Maxim's, you just don't get seated where we're sitting
unless you're fabulously rich, a huge celebrity, a government minister, or a sheik. So that's Maxim's. Now you
tell me how you all got seated in this room, especially in
those perfectly awful clothes." Another muffled laugh.

That I could tell her. It had been just one more of
Michael's little masterpieces. He never did anything halfway, particularly where public entertainments were involved. If Maxim's was where you were supposed to be,
that is where he and his friends would be, and, by God,
royally seated. And, as in the conduct of his business, no

detail of advance planning would be overlooked. A month before the trip, Michael had called Pierre, the young French proprietor of one of San Francisco's most exclusive restaurants. Pierre had trained and worked at Maxim's for years before opening his own place in the States, and had retained close ties with his former employer. He had learned his lessons well in Paris, since his San Francisco restaurant's pretentious ambience, its humorless and arrogant staff, the mediocrity of its food, and the character and motives of its clientele comprised virtually a mirror image, albeit in miniature, of Yolaine's description of Maxim's. Michael spent a small fortune every year with Pierre, so he had no qualms about asking him for a favor — to make the arrangements with Maxim's, ensure that his French colleagues understood the importance of the people and the event, and guarantee our royal reception.

So Maxim's had prepared for the best — an august group of Chicago bankers, wealthy San Francisco entrepreneurs, and the customary sprinkling of Japanese financiers. When what they got turned out to be not the best, but the *worst* — a motley grab bag of disheveled poachers — they had no alternative but to try to make do with the horrible hand they had been dealt.

There were three tables set in the place of honor along the dance floor — our two, and a third that remained unoccupied for an hour or so. About ten o'clock, the other celebrated party arrived. If we had thought the staff's dyspepsia a bit overwrought, at least one good reason for it swept into the room in all its forbidding glory — Christina Onassis and entourage. In tow behind the frumpy heiress were a gorgeous statuesque blonde and four or five very large, very dark, very menacing creatures in black ties. Miss Onassis said something to one of her larger black-tied escorts, who in turn said something to the maître d', who — now ashen-faced — shrugged helplessly, shook his head, and babbled a response that I assumed to be an obsequious apology for our presence and a sworn assurance that never again would Miss Onassis be subjected to such an insufferable indignity. The maître d' bowed several times in a cowed retreat. The escort shot a black glance at our table, which I returned with a nod and a cavalier smile. And there we were ensconced in the center room of Maxim's — just me and my friends, and Christina and hers.

As for Yolaine, she wasn't at all interested in the Onassis party's problems. For several minutes she had been lost in concentration, creating a huge, trembling pyramid out of the twelve champagne glasses that she had collected from around the table. Most of the glasses were at least half-full and, if the elegant structure were to fall, it would mean chaos and, most likely, the gendarmes. Everyone at the table was afraid to breathe, the two hovering waiters were paralyzed, and the captain was a vision of speechless fury. The edifice completed, Yolaine carefully examined it from all angles, smiled her satisfaction, and then — with a swift flick of her hand — removed a glass from the very center of the stack. By all known laws of physics, the structure should have collapsed in an explosion of splashing champagne and shattering glass, but, by some magic, it remained proudly erect. From the tables of the proletariat, out somewhere beyond the royal circle, there came an eruption of laughter, applause, and bravos. In acknowledgment, Yolaine demurely raised the glass in the direction of her admirers, drank it dry, and then held it out to the livid captain. "Oh, monsieur, as you can see the glass is empty. Would you kindly pour a little more, please?" He did as he was bid and, furious but thoroughly intimidated, stomped off. The Onassis party, upstaged by the girl from the visiting circus, sulked.

It was that kind of night.

We danced through the night, wildly to the fast music and tenderly to the slow, exchanged bad jokes, laughed, and drank champagne. At midnight Yolaine suggested that we move on to Harry's Bar, which everybody did, since she was now in charge. There, we searched for the ghosts of an earlier generation of American romantics wonderfully lost in Paris, and, finding none, settled for bourbon, cognac, and any other liquids that were at hand. Yolaine and I held hands and giggled and touched each other's cheeks with our fingertips. Later, with the night slipping away, we made tender and passionate love in the tiny, sparsely furnished garret that I had managed to extract from the overbooked Ritz. In the morning, I apologized for the meagerness of the room. Stretching her slender bare body before an open window and drinking the cool air, she told me it was the most romantic room in the world. I joined her at the window, we looked out over the slate rooftops and chimneys of Paris, and I saw that she was right. We each felt, but did not mention, the approaching bittersweet end of the dream. I asked her when she had to go home, and she said late afternoon, and we decided we should have lunch together away from the crowd. She called her friend Henri Faucheron, and he gave us a secluded corner and had us served with a minimum of staff intrusion. We had so little time to learn about each other but, even with our imminent return to our respective worlds, felt compelled to know all we could. We had to know that our time together was as important as we thought it was. She said that she loved to ski, asked if I was a good skier, and I lied that I was. I told her that I loved tennis, and she lied that she did too. She wanted to know if I believed in God, and I honestly replied that I did, but probably not in the way most people did. She said she was a Catholic but, having studied meditational disciplines in an ashram in the south of France, she was also a Buddhist. I told her it was not possible to be both a believing Christian and a Buddhist, and she let my presumption pass. She wanted to know about my former wife and my daughters, and I told her that I loved them. She told me that she had a lover who was married, to whom she had always been faithful, and that she had at first felt guilty about her infidelity in being with me. I was angry and jealous and told her that it was philosophically impossible to be unfaithful to a man who was cheating on his wife. She let that presumption pass too, although not without a quizzical look that asked whether I understood anything at all about life. She delicately changed the subject, asked about my education, and I told her about Yale. She took her degree in economics at the University of Paris. And we were happy to know that we shared not only passion but a modicum of intellect. Her father was le Comte de Bernard du Briel, aristocrat; mine was Thomas L. Smart, very good insurance salesman. She had two sisters, a niece, and nephew. I had two brothers, three sisters, and twenty-odd nieces and nephews. She was not a good swimmer and neither was I. We both liked oysters, sardines, and ripe cheese.

We sat silently for a long time, playing with our desserts with our forks but not eating. At the same instant we suddenly looked up from our plates into each other's eyes and, in perfect unison, said, "I love you." The wonderful shock of the moment brought both laughter and unashamed tears. While the heady circumstances of our high-octane romance might have had the appearance of a "fling," at that moment we knew that this was not coy play-acting, but an awesome commitment of souls.

She was twenty-five and I was forty-six. We never gave it a thought. To me, she had the wisdom and life force of a queen of a thousand years. And, to her, I was a pillar of ageless strength and trustworthiness who would elevate her spirit and open the doors to self-fulfillment.

What she did not then know, and neither did I, was that she was pledging her love, and entrusting her thirst for life, to a middle-aged drug addict. The sickness was not yet plain even to me.

If I didn't fully realize that the Faucheron lunch had sealed my future, it was crystal clear that it at least required an immediate amendment of my short-term plans. Egypt suddenly had no importance, and I asked Yolaine how she would feel if I canceled that leg of the trip and returned to Teildras for a week as a hotel guest. She was as ecstatic at the prospect as I, so we laid plans for my return, which required a small conspiracy.

As I had surmised, the father had a tendency to become outraged over his daughters' affairs of the flesh — particularly where his youngest, and favorite, was concerned. If I was to reappear, it must look like an arm's-length transaction — simply a former dinner guest, having fallen in love with the place, returning for a week's lodgings.

The sisters would drive back that evening. In the morning, Carole, who ordinarily took reservations, would report the nice American's phone call from Paris to request a room. Yolaine would meet the six-thirty train in Angers and drive the nice American to the château. There could be no hint of the Paris affair or, indeed, that a rendezvous, however innocent, had ever occurred there. Yolaine had gone to Paris on the pretext of a wisdom tooth that required attention; and Carole, they told her mother, had to go along in case Yolaine was too ill to drive back. Acquiring a lover had not been on the purported agenda.

We could take our meals together, visit with the family in the salon, go for walks in the woods, and maybe even spend an afternoon in town; all of which, after a couple of days, would appear to be no more than the graceful ripening of a natural friendship, and not a cause for alarm. There could, of course, be no thought of intimacy; to be discovered in flagrante delicto would surely precipitate a paternal fury best avoided.

156

The arrangement didn't bother me; indeed, it was I who first suggested it. Considering the direction our relationship was taking, I needed to gain her family's respect, and the last thing I wanted to do was to insult her father by ravishing his daughter under his own roof. So we swore to be celibate for a week.

"Papa," she said, "I'm sure you remember Mr. Smart. He was with the American group that we enjoyed so much last week."

"Of course. I'm delighted to have you back for a longer visit."

"I had such a lovely time that evening, with your kindness and the beauty of your house, that I couldn't leave France without coming back here to relax for a few days."

"I am very pleased, monsieur. How was the train from Paris?"

"Well, a train is a train, but yours are much better than ours. It was a pleasant trip."

"Good. Let me show you your room. You can freshen up and, if you like, we can have a drink before dinner." Le Comte picked up my three bags, one of them very heavy, and, without losing a breath, led me up two flights of stairs and into one of the loveliest rooms I had ever seen. I marveled at this strong old man — displaced aristocrat forced to play innkeeper, sommelier, porter, and, I would learn, an assortment of other menial roles; yet the very soul of self-respect. I wondered if I would ever know him. I wanted to; I loved his daughter.

He and I sat for a while in the salon sipping drinks and talking politics. He told me that Giscard was good for France and that Carter was bad for the world. I told him I couldn't comment about Giscard but agreed with him on Carter. He asked me why Americans had permitted the media to destroy the great Nixon, who, in the European view, was the most effective American President of

157

this century. I tried to explain that Americans have this thing about the *way* things are done, that, regardless of a person's brilliance as a statesman, we do not suffer flagrant crooks gladly. He told me that that is both Americans' charm and their flaw — their hopelessly naïve innocence of life — and I allowed as how that might be so. It was evident that he respected me and had not an inkling that I had laid lustful hands on his daughter. In that, I was glad for myself, but — with a sentiment that surprised me — I was even gladder for him.

There were few guests that night, and Yolaine told her mother that since I was alone, she thought it would be a gracious thing for her to have dinner with the nice American. Her mother said that was a fine idea and commended Yolaine for her thoughtfulness. We sat separated by a small table, drinking champagne, looking dreamily into each other's eyes, saying very little and playing with each other's feet under the table. I asked Yolaine to tell me about her father. "Oh, some other time!" she said impatiently. "I'm feeling very romantic and just want to look at you." That was a lie; she was caressing my ankle with her foot in a willful act of exquisite torture, and delighting in her perversity. "No, now," I said, and brought both feet back under my chair and locked my knees together like a maiden resisting deflowerment.

"All right. Papa is the last directly descended male of a very old and once-rich family. This elegant little country hotel you see is not, to him, just a hotel. It is his house — his *family* house. My mother and he made it into a hotel to keep from losing it. If they had lost it, Papa would have died — literally. The house is so much of his identity — a tie to a world his mother told him about when he was a child, a world that she made him believe was *his* world, even though it was dying even then. And today, the hotel operation gives him self-respect at a time when he's incapable of doing much else. Incapable not because of stupidity — he is a brilliant man — but because his crazy mother basically prepared him to be a counselor to Bonaparte, who inconveniently died long before Papa was born.

"When I was a little girl, we still had money. I don't know how much, but I think a lot. We lived in Paris. Mama was the most beautiful woman in the city, and Papa was probably the handsomest man in all of France — actually, he still is. Don't you think so? There were stories that we had once been even richer, but, through some dumb business decisions during the war, his family had lost valuable hotel properties in Paris. But, whatever that had been about, we still lived in great luxury. I thought I was a princess. In those days, Teildras was our country house. We would come down from Paris for Christmas and Easter holidays and on weekends in the summer. The place is so huge that the two wings were closed off, and we only used the main house. We had no electricity then — can you imagine that? There were huge candelabras for light. Every room had a fireplace, and Papa kept them all full of burning logs. Christmas was *fantastic!* Papa and Mama would have a lot of their friends over. The men would shoot birds — we had a lot more land then — and we had incredible feasts. We had a huge tree, and Mama filled every part of the house with the most beautiful decorations you can imagine."

Glancing around a room that was full of priceless antiques and tapestries, and even in June warmed by a crackling fire, it was easy for me to imagine those years. The scene wasn't too different now from what it must have been then — the only changes were the addition of the small dinner tables and the electric chandeliers and, of course, the paying guests instead of family and old friends.

"But what did your father *do* then — I mean, when he wasn't hunting game or entertaining?" I asked.

"You don't understand. He never really had a regular

job, as far as I know. His mother — who really was quite addled by the time I knew her, strutting around here in clothes from, God, I don't know what century, playing the grande dame and making life miserable for Mama — had this crazy idea that aristocrats aren't supposed to work. That was the responsibility of peasants, coal miners, and bourgeois shopkeepers. Aristocrats are supposed to *preside*. And that's mostly what Papa did. Can you believe that — in this century? A son educated *not* to work? Except, of course, for his years as a naval officer. *Grande-mère* thought that was okay for aristocrats."

I learned that when the de Bernards lived in Paris, Le Comte apparently spent most of his time at his men's club — where he and his buddies sat around and talked about politics and investments and the country club. One year he was the French amateur golf champion. Yolaine also told me that her father was a naturally gifted architect who had designed a few houses for friends and a major golf course, even though he had never had any training. But his talents obviously didn't include making money. He'd had a lot of it from his family, and became an easy target for his so-called buddies at the club. On their advice, he made a few small investments. Then they came up with a fabulous project in Latin America that would earn him a fortune. Le Comte put all his money into it; the promoter disappeared and so did the money.

The story seemed so much at odds with the aura of dignity and self-assurance that surrounded the man that I had to hear more. "Go on, sweetheart, what happened then?"

"Papa was sixty years old and had no idea how to make a living. We had to leave Paris and come here to live. But it would only be a matter of time before we would lose this place too. The income from the tenant farmer was barely enough to pay the taxes. That would have finished

Papa, and Mama wasn't going to let it happen. Papa had no money but he still had his good name, and Mama had a plan. He was able to pledge the property and get a big bank loan for renovation. The first floor of the main house was partitioned into these two dining rooms and the large salon, the two upper floors were made into eleven suites, and a restaurant kitchen was installed. We opened up the west wing, which had been closed for probably a century, and made some very simple apartments for the family to live in — there wasn't enough money, and there still isn't enough, to make them nice.

"Papa did every bit of the architectural design himself and Mama did the decorating. I think you probably find your apartment quite elegant. Well, that's Mama's work, all of it. She has the most exquisite taste in the world.

"So, all of a sudden, there we all were in the hotel business — without a bit of experience."

"Well, experience or not, from what I see around me it looks as though your parents have made the place an extraordinary success," I said.

Yolaine laughed. "Well, that depends on how you define success. Every year is a grinding financial struggle. But a success in their minds; and a success in the minds of the clients — yes, in that sense, Teildras is a fabulous success, the finest place of its size, with the best cuisine in all of France. Catherine Deneuve comes to Teildras. Lord Carrington comes to Teildras for his vacations. And now, with *your* help, my dear, Paul Newman comes here. It's that kind of place. And you know why? It isn't just the house and the food; it's *them* — Mama and Papa, their charm and grace and dignity."

I knew what she was talking about. Those qualities, and the pride. I had felt them at once. Teildras, the exquisite country hotel, while a necessity of family survival, was, in their minds, merely a logical extension — appropriately modified for the times — of Teildras, the four-hundred-year-old manor first owned by the Bishop of Anjou, and then the house of generations of de Bernards.

Yolaine asked whether I'd noticed the portrait of the beautiful woman in the reception area. "Now *there* is an authentic de Bernard tradition for you. She's Charlotte — the reason we all exist, and Papa worships her. During the Jacobin terror they had a novel way of killing aristocrats in Anjou. They loaded everybody into boats, took them out into the middle of the Loire, and drowned them. Charlotte was, I think, four or five years old, and the last survivor of the family. A servant woman who was determined to save her cut off Charlotte's hair and disguised her as a peasant boy. Another time, she hid the little girl under her skirt. Charlotte grew up, married another aristocrat after the Revolution had faded away, had children, and is the de Bernard family heroine.

"Do you believe that story? I do. But the important thing is that Papa does. He's been driven to keep the house for his daughters and future generations; but I think he has done it as much for Charlotte. Sometimes, I wonder if he thinks *I'm* Charlotte." The touch of irony in her voice as she said it was outweighed by the affection. "Oh, Papa reveres the past, but I'll tell you this — these days, he's living very much with the realities of the present. Every day from March to the end of November, he and Mama are up at seven and work until midnight. *Every day*, seven days a week! Mama is in the kitchen, preparing sauces and cooking, supervising one or two helpers. Papa is buying vegetables and fish in town and carrying luggage and entertaining guests and getting wine from the cave and trying to make sense of the books, for which he has no head at all. *And he is seventy years old and she is sixty-seven!*

"Why do they do it? Certainly not for money. There *still* is no money. Almost every year, Papa has to sell off a little more land. My parents are running the loveliest little hotel in France and, for all their work, they'll never be free of debt. Unless they sell, which they will never do. They'll just keep doing what they are doing every day of every week until they can't manage it anymore. They'll do it because of love and family and dignity. And because they're *le Comte et la Comtesse de Bernard du Breil.*"

I thought of the first time I had seen the mother, when James and I had barged into the kitchen barely a week earlier at one o'clock in the morning — a small sinewy woman, perfectly coiffed, wearing an elegant black dress accented by white pearls, cleaning up a sink. And now, I was quite without words.

"Well, you insisted that I tell you about my father. I guess you got more than you asked for — the whole god-damn de Bernard melodrama." She was almost whispering, her face flushed and her eyes wet. She bit hard on the end of her thumb to keep her jaw from trembling. I had fallen in love with a carefree, comic, glamorous girl — the toast of Maxim's; a girl of laughter who could work magic with champagne glasses, and make love with hot passion and exquisite tenderness. Only a day later I was not with a different woman, but certainly a more complete one, who had just revealed to me the whole of her life — which was not to be confused with a blissful night of Parisian fantasy. I was again with the girl in the baggy green dress, serving drinks and food to hotel guests; only on that first night — which now seemed years ago — I hadn't given a thought to what it meant. In her telling of her parents' story, I knew that she had been telling her own — a cultured child of nobility, raised with reverence for her heritage, educated in the best schools, with the world before her for the taking, suddenly reduced to waiting on tables in service to the family honor. A story told not with bitterness, but with her own fierce, burning pride.

For the first time, I took conscious note of the tapestries, with their lavish but fading portrayals of chivalrous love, religious devotionals, and ancient battles for glory. I looked at my woman — this marvelous amalgam of frivolity, loyalty, and fierceness — and loved her with a love that eclipsed any emotion I had ever known in my life. I knew she would be in my future and, naïvely, I wanted to be in her past. I wanted to be a part of the tapestry, mounted on a white charger with lance held high, her father riding beside me, to do battle with infidels. Yolaine's intensity had left me not only deeply loving, but also with a rising agitation. I excused myself from the table.

I sat on the toilet and fumbled around in my jacket pocket to find the vial. I took a couple of good hits and in a few seconds felt the glow — at once relaxed and recharged. I wondered what Yolaine would think if she knew about the cocaine. At Maxim's, during a rambling conversation about everything and nothing, I had slipped in an innocent question about how she felt about drugs. Her response had not been encouraging. She had spent six months as the receptionist and bookkeeper at Ma Maison in Beverly Hills a couple of years earlier and, having fallen in with a fast crowd in and around the film business, had fooled around with pot and "a couple of other things." I asked her if cocaine was one of them, and she said that she had had a little, but finding the L.A. drug scene, and all that went with it, disgusting, she had pulled out of it before she got herself into trouble. She hated drugs and the people who used them. I had thought about telling her how cocaine was different from the really dangerous drugs, how all of the best people were using it, and how, taken in moderation, it could be a nice experience; I had wanted to get her on the same wave length with me for the night. But, considering the strength of her feelings, I had thought better of it. Tonight wasn't the right occasion either. For now, all she would know was that her new lover had limitless energy, great humor, and a gift for eloquence; she could learn the magic for herself in her own good time.

A little more cocaine put me into deep thought about the fabulous history of Yolaine's family and their present situation. They were all so full of a love for life, and for each other. I had missed something in my own family; and, whatever it was, I was sure I would find it here.

Inadvertently, that week, Yolaine and I let our love slip out of the closet and, with our public flaunting of it, the tension in the great old house had become as taut as an overstrung bow. Sometimes, when Le Comte de Bernard came into the dining room at lunchtime and saw us holding hands across the table, immersed in each other's eyes and intently whispered words, I felt as though the air was congealing into mud and that, unless I could escape into the outdoors, I surely would suffocate. And the pressure of his outraged will was all the more threatening for its relentless silence.

My first night in the house, Yolaine had said to hell with our pact of temporary celibacy, and, despite my protests that it wasn't wise, had come to my room to make love and sleep. To my amazement, she had confided in her mother and, with her mother's complicity, a supposedly foolproof scheme had been concocted to keep her father happily ignorant. The plan proved to be neither foolproof nor even very smart in theory, and the old man discovered the tryst with the sunrise. I was spared a direct confrontation, which at the time I mistook as a sign of mercy, but he read Yolaine the riot act — whorish behavior, outraged family dignity, a personal insult, and all of that. And her concise response, barren of even pro forma remorse, was even more infuriating to him than the carnal act itself. "Papa, I'm sorry you feel that way, but you really don't understand. I love Richard. I intend to sleep with him, and it really is none of your affair."

He had not spoken a word to me that fateful morning nor any day since. Not even a "good morning" when I descended the stairs for breakfast. When we passed in the hallways and couldn't avoid an encounter, his eyes looked straight through me. It was an unpropitious beginning with a potential father-in-law. I took to spending most of my daytimes reading in my room.

Given the direction my relationship with Yolaine was taking, I desperately wanted some conversation with her father; an old-fashioned man-to-man talk about how true my love was, how worthy my intentions were, and what a good, responsible son-in-law I would be. But Yolaine cautioned me against overtures that would be taken as a sign of weakness and badly received. "Papa really had no choice in any of this. Let matters take their course, give him time to accept the idea, and he'll eventually come around on his own. Nothing you say now is going to make a difference, anyway. He's a proud, stubborn man, and he thinks he's been wounded. He'll recover, but you've got to let him make the first move."

Despite the anxiety, the evenings were full of laughter, wine, and romance. At dinner, the dining room was filled with happy guests, and Yolaine and I could lose ourselves in a dimly lit corner for hours of *foie gras*, duck, fine Bordeaux, and desserts graced with champagne. Carole, as she attended to the needs of guests, would sneak a few moments here and there to sip wine with us and reminisce about our wild Paris night and her key role in the conspiracy of our love. And each evening, as midnight approached and with her work finished in the kitchen, Yolaine's mother would join us for coffee. The mother and daughter would chat away in French, now solemnly, now with a chuckle; here an arched eyebrow and a shrug, there a mock frown and a spreading of the hands.

Yolaine would give me an occasional translation, but even without the help it was easy to figure out the subject of these nightly mother-daughter conversations — *l'affaire de Richard et Yolaine*. La Comtesse de Bernard had no more use for me than did her husband, but her feminine instinct dictated a totally different response. Where he reacted out of the wounded male ego of an insulted father, she, no doubt with memories of her own first great romance, immediately became her daughter's confidante, calmly sympathizing with her impassioned state, offering gentle words of caution and reason.

But La Comtesse's benign air was born of more than sympathy; the handsome old woman knew that the more adamant the parental opposition to the outrageous affair, the more intent her strong-headed daughter would be in pursuing it to its predictably ignominious end. She herself had once been a spirited young girl in Paris, working in the glittering world of haute couture and exposed to all the adventures that went with it, and she understood the futility of a father's outrage. Besides, all three of her daughters had always been careless of conventions, and her youngest, in the forthright certitude with which she pursued her impulses, had always been the least amenable to parental interferences.

No, La Comtesse was sure that it would be better to forgo angry protests and dire warnings, and just let this particular passion of the moment wear itself out — as surely it would. I knew that had been her thinking when she had unsuccessfully conspired in the scheme to get Yolaine into my room without her father's knowledge. And I knew it was her thinking as she sat with us at table, playing with her dessert, sipping coffee, chatting away with her daughter, and occasionally tossing me a wry but not unkind glance, indulging in her nightly ritual of feigned goodwill just prior to the hour when she knew that her daughter and I would retreat to my room for another night of passion. "Don't make any big scenes," I could imagine her telling herself. "The American will be leaving in a couple of days, and this great romance soon will tire of its own weight, reduced to a pleasant memory of an adventurous fling that my daughter will smile over in her later years."

It was good strategy. But La Comtesse didn't understand the intensity of our love. And neither she nor I grasped the single-mindedness of her daughter's new purpose. The morning of the day before my scheduled departure, Yolaine told me that she had decided to return with me to the United States for a few days. "If we're going to be married, it's important that I know something about your life," she said. "I want to see how you live in your country, and be with you there — now."

That was an announcement I wasn't prepared for. I had promised to return to France at the end of the summer, after getting my business affairs in order and making some money. Then, we could begin to plan our future seriously. But my love intended to come with me, and that was that.

Our relationship had been all quick passion, champagne, and laughter; elegant restaurants, an exclusive hotel, and a country château out of a storybook; dancing till dawn in Paris and making love through soft summer nights. She didn't want to close the carnival down.

We had never known each other as real people in a real world, and I was as afraid as she was that, if we turned off the music too quickly, in our period of separation we might forget the tune.

I had felt strongly that, precisely because of the intensity of our passion, our love would benefit from a period of retreat. But the overriding reason for my reluctance to take her with me was, quite simply, that I was fast running out of cash. Such a trip would be the height of irresponsibility. I just couldn't afford it.

Yolaine and I had never discussed money. She had seen me only in atmospheres of profligate spending, surrounded by rich friends, merrily indulging in the pleasures of Paris with an openhanded outpouring of American dollars that said, more eloquently than words, "Price is no object." I didn't want to mislead her, but neither was it the right time for disillusionment. For the time being, I thought it better not to say anything about being financially strapped. If it occurred to me that silence itself could be a lie, the thought passed quickly.

So I gave her a safer and, I thought, persuasive argument. "Look, sweetheart, you know how much I love you, and there isn't anything in the world I'd rather do than run off with you right now and forever. But I'm not going directly back to San Francisco, you know. I'm flying to Washington to do some work for some clients. I'm going to be back here in a couple of months anyway, and, in the meantime, I'm hoping your father might start to believe that this relationship is based on something other than craziness. Your going off with me now won't help."

"So you're going to Washington," she said. "I would *love* to see Washington. That's as much your world as San Francisco, isn't it? You can work all day long if you have to; I'll keep busy visiting museums and monuments. And we'll have our nights together. And maybe we could have a day or two in New York. As for Papa, he's already as angry as he can get. I'll be gone only for a week or so, and when I return he'll be all the better for it."

"Well, it's certainly worth thinking about," I said in a studied tone of noncommitment. "I think I'll go up to the room for a fast nap before lunch."

As I started up the stairs, the last words I heard were a gaily tossed-off "Then it's settled, *mon amour?*"

I hadn't the faintest idea how I could manage such a trip, and by the time I reached my room I was in a nervous sweat. It was clear that I would either have to take Yolaine with me or think up a believable excuse, other than money, for leaving her behind. And the excuse route didn't hold much promise, since my ebullient new love had a marked gift for arguing the implausible into absolute reasonableness — a task made easier for her by my reluctance to deny her anything and thus tarnish my image.

I had a little over a gram of coke left. My measured use of the drug during the week at Teildras had served me well, just the right amount to keep me wired enough to be amusing at dinner and, despite the exhausting hours we kept, competent in bed, without pushing me into nervous agitation. I could have a little now, a little more around dinnertime, and, if I was careful, enough would be left to get me nicely through the long flight from Paris to Washington. But I'd have to call my friend Congressman X, and restock as soon as I got to town. Oh God, that was a cost I hadn't factored into my calculations — one that I'd have whether Yolaine went with me or not; at least five or six hundred dollars' worth of the stuff to support ten days or so of a heavy schedule of work and play while I was in the East. Well, that could be handled with an additional overdraft. The purchase couldn't really be called an extravagant luxury; it was a necessity of the pace of life.

I dipped my miniature spoon twice into the vial, took a small snort up each nostril, and walked to the window to think some more. The fatigue and anxiety vanished. The green of the meadow and blue of the sky took on a new richness, and the puffs of clouds drifting in from Brittany billowed round and voluptuous. La Comtesse's flowers in the courtyard outdid themselves with radiant color. And my refreshed and reenlightened brain created a scenario that would work.

Of *course* Yolaine would go with me; suddenly it made a great deal of sense. In Washington, I had an open account at the Madison. I could sign for the room and whatever meals we took in the Montpelier Room. Unlike most hotel restaurants, its food was excellent, and Yolaine would love the paneling and the chandeliers. I had a past-due bill of about three thousand dollars, but that wouldn't be a problem. The Madison had become my home away from home. I had been spending over ten thousand dollars a year there and had become a favored guest at Washington's headquarters of power, money, and elegance. The Madison would not only help solve my cash problems; its solicitous treatment of us would impress Yolaine no end.

And in New York we'd get our shelter at the Sherry-Netherland. I was past-due there too, but not badly, and I was confident that I could bluff my way through any embarrassment, and get away with a signature on the bill. The Sherry-Netherland wasn't the Pierre; but, frequented by California show business moguls and agents, it had a nouveau riche panache that Yolaine would find amusing. Located on New York's hottest intersection, across from the Plaza and Central Park, it also happened to be where I had an account; there weren't alternatives even if I wanted to consider any.

Yes, Yolaine's idea was brilliant! It had scared me off at first, but any difficulties could be surmounted with a little planning, and it was a wonderful chance to combine business and pleasure. While in Washington, I would make a few calls on congressmen, drop by to see Senator Cranston, and meet with somebody at the Department of Transportation — a little bit of casual lobbying that would justify billing my Philadelphia and San Francisco clients for expense reimbursement and consulting fees. And, in New York, I'd have a meeting or two with the people at the Port Authority. That would get me reimbursement of most of my expenses for that leg of the trip and some more fees. All in all, I figured to come out of the week netting maybe five thousand dollars after paying Yolaine's expenses and buying some coke. I wouldn't be able to do much about the bank loan and the overdrafts for a few months, but *priorities* would be handled okay. And we would have a marvelous time.

I picked up the room phone, got the overseas operator, and reached Betty at the Madison. The Madison was routinely "full" when a stranger called for reservations; but, even calling at the last minute, I could always get one of the few rooms they held back for special people. She asked whether I wanted my usual accommodation. "No," I told her, "I think I'll take one of your suites." It was, after all, a special occasion.

I could hardly wait to tell Yolaine the news.

Yolaine didn't need to be told; by the time I joined her for lunch, she had already advised her mother that she was going with me. I thought her action outrageously presumptuous but let it pass; I was too much in love to quibble, and we were both elated at my confirmation of her insistent plan.

"What did your mother say?" Given the mother's decent demeanor toward me, I had reason to hope for understanding if not a blessing.

"She said, *'Mon Dieu, tu es absolument folle.'* "

"Don't be funny," I said. "What about your father?"

"He doesn't know yet. Mama's going to tell him."

"Oh great, just absolutely great," I said in undisguised despair. "The two of them already detest me. I really don't know how I'm going to get through another day and night in this house. I do hope you made it clear that this whole thing is your idea and that I'm not just absconding with their precious daughter."

Her cheeks suddenly flushed. "Oh good Jesus, you're my *man*, aren't you? Well *act* like my man! Papa's bigger than you and probably stronger than you, but he's seventy years old, after all; I'm sure that, if you're fast enough, you can beat him in a fight." Her pique passed and she burst into laughter, squeezed my arm, and blew me a kiss. "Come on, it's all going to be okay; you'll see. Just be a little tough."

After dinner Le Comte came to the table, standing very tall and looking very solemn. "Richard," he said, "I think we should have a talk."

"I would like that very much," I said. "I've been wanting to talk to you for several days, but it's been impossible." And, anxious to preempt the emotional field before he had a chance to fire even a short salvo, I launched into a compulsive monologue.

"I know that none of this looks good to you. But I want you to understand that I love Yolaine. I'm not just some cavalier adventurer having a quick affair with your daughter." Yolaine stifled a giggle. "I'm very serious. In fact, we think we want to get married." I worried that I was breathing too fast.

"I know that isn't a big comfort to you now, since you know nothing about me. And I'm aware that Yolaine's impetuous. Well, I'm not. This has been a fast romance, I know that. But we aren't going to rush into marriage. This trip to the States is nothing more than an extended period for getting to know each other better, and it's Yolaine's idea, not mine." True or not, Yolaine was disgusted by the cowardly disclaimer and she shot me a withering glance that said so. "She'll be back in little more than a week, I promise you that." He looked skeptical.

"Moreover, I promise you that, if we do marry, it won't be for at least a year. I've got enough sense to know that we're from very different worlds, and we've got to take the time to be sure of what we're doing." I heard my words running out in a torrent of unseemly supplication, and was embarrassed at my own sounds.

"And, please, understand how sorry I am about what has occurred in this house. It hasn't been my intention to insult you in your own home; I've nothing but respect for Yolaine, for you, and your family. It's just that we're very much in love."

It sounded lame and mushy even to me, and, in search of approval, I stole a glance at Yolaine, sitting across the table by her father. Her lips were tightly drawn and she quickly, almost imperceptibly, shook her head from side to side. She had warned me never to apologize to her father for anything, and certainly not for making love to his daughter, at Teildras or anyplace else. She was a grown woman, it was her house as much as his, she would damn well do what she liked there, and that was that.

There was a big silence, and I felt compelled to fill it. "And I want you to know that I'll take care of Yolaine and treat her with great respect. I believe in fidelity in marriage; I'll be faithful to her." I realized that I was babbling on, reaching for any noble cliché I could dredge up, in a mistaken belief that saccharine sentimentality could prove character.

The old man had sat through my monologue with a face of impassive resolve, his expression not varying a whit — until he heard that last statement. One bushy eyebrow arched and one corner of the finely carved mouth raised ever so slightly, clearly asking, "Are you crazy, or what?" As often as not among the French upper crust, "social" marriages were entered into out of consideration of money, property, position, and the parties' mutual ambitions; it was, of course, necessary that they like each other, and if by chance they loved out of a deep passion, so much the better; if not, they could each take their pleasure with others without the world falling apart. For a time, it might be obligatory for me to massage his daughter with such romantic nonsense, but *he* certainly didn't want to hear it; it was utterly irrelevant to his concerns.

I had run out of platitudes, which was just as well since I had a feeling that I had played the fool. Sensing that I

174

was exhausted of romantic chatter, he took a sip of wine and went after the facts.

"Are you Catholic?"

"No."

"Well, *we are*."

"That's fine with me. I've nothing against Catholicism; in fact I've often thought in recent years that, if I ever felt an urge for a church again, Catholicism might be my choice."

"I understand you are divorced."

"That's right."

"There hasn't been a divorce in the de Bernard family in four hundred years."

"Well, I'm sorry to break the record. Perhaps it would be more satisfactory if I weren't divorced and, in deference to Continental customs, took your daughter for my mistress instead of my wife." That brought me a very dark look, but no rejoinder.

"You're much older than Yolaine."

"Yes, I am."

"How much older?"

"Twenty years."

"That's a lot. That age difference can lead to problems."

"Yes, it can. But we know that whatever time we have together, whether it's five years or fifty years, it's going to be a lot more rewarding than most couples ever know, whatever their ages." This time I thought I saw a softening in the eyes and the hint of a smile.

"What about children?"

"We hope to have some."

"Will they be Catholic or Protestant?"

"Frankly, I don't give a damn. I don't think churches should fight for the ownership of children any more than I think parents should." I was proud of that one, but if he caught its thrust he was not nonplussed by it.

"And will they be French or American? Yolaine is French, you know — *very* French."

Ah, I thought, there it was — the emotional bottom line. Le Comte was mightily concerned about the practicalities of this potential marriage, but, transcending all of that, was the fact of heritage. I had learned that, however much they loved to squabble among themselves, French families had a marvelous closeness. Against the rest of the world, they were bastions of fierce loyalty. And, with all the tensions between them, it was clear that Yolaine was her father's cherished favorite. Although headstrong, and often a thorn painfully stuck in his sensibilities, the youngest and brightest of his daughters was the most valued possession of this proud old man who would have no sons. Despite their skirmishes, he saw in her the continuity of generations of aristocracy and family and Frenchness, the child most competent in mind, sentiment, and will to protect and nourish the tradition.

And now it looked as though she was about to run off to a life of hot dogs and plastic plates in a country that, for all the hectic melodrama of its brief life, hadn't as much real tradition and historical depth as abided in his single household.

"Look," I said, "it's important that you understand something. I love Yolaine for who and what she *is* — what she is *right now*. And what she is is French, and your daughter, and the product of the whole history of your family. *That's* whom I love. I love her and the culture that produced her. I don't want to make her into something else — to Americanize her. I want her to spend a lot of time here every year, hopefully with me with her, soaking up more and more of this wonderful culture and being part of the small, civilized world that you and your family have created here. As for the children, they'll be *your* grandchildren, and they'll be as much French as American."

"You don't even speak French," he said; he had been trying to be decent toward me, but no amount of studied niceness could conceal the contempt in his words. "You can't understand the French people if you don't understand the language. Our character and the feel of our culture is in our language. You can't know us in translation."

I knew there was a grain of truth in what he said, but the point had been made to me too many times — by Yolaine, her sister, and half-a-dozen other Frenchmen — and it was getting tiresome. Plus, the French exaggerated it to the brink of boorishness. I loved the sound of the language, and it obviously expressed something special about its proprietors that transcended the communication of literal meanings. But I had trouble regarding it as the country's most precious national resource, or as the currency of an arcane exclusivity, inaccessible to culturally deprived foreigners.

"I'll learn it," I said, "although I think I understand Yolaine quite well as it is." There was just enough sarcasm, I thought, to implicitly dismiss his arrogance, and just the right touch of a subtle message that I would be the winner in any contest over his daughter, linguistic ignoramus or not.

Le Comte indicated that the audience was over. "Well," he said, "I'm not happy about any of this, but I believe you're sincere, if badly misguided. Time will tell. We'll just have to see what happens." He was as fatigued as I. With a face turned gray but still possessed of every taut line of its dignity, he excused himself and went to bed.

We had our luggage packed and loaded into Carole's car early the next morning. She would drive us to the station, we would take the train to Paris and spend the night before our flight to Washington at la Residence du Bois, an elegant little hotel just off avenue Foch.

Le Comte came out to the parking area, said a few words to Yolaine, kissed her on the cheek, nodded to me, and went back into the house. He wasn't about to dignify our departure with an excess of ceremony. La Comtesse, who had busied herself since dawn preparing a good breakfast and helping Yolaine pack, hovered around the car till the very end.

With all the logistical work done, there was nothing left but the hardest part — mother's and daughter's good-byes, whispered words of counsel, and tears. While that went on, I stood a few yards apart, feeling like a huge weed in a flower garden and, for the first time, a little guilty, drawing circles in the gravel with my foot, smoking cigarettes, and pretending to stare at some compelling object on the far horizon. Finally, unable to take it any longer, I went over to the two women and took Yolaine gently by the arm.

"Look, my love, your mother's got to understand how serious I am, how much you mean to me. Remind her that, when I first got to France, I had intended to go on to Egypt on some important business, and that because of my love for you — and *only* because of my love — I canceled those plans. Just to be with you — and to get to know your family. That should mean something to her."

Yolaine translated my message, and the older woman replied with a solemnity of tone that I felt sure meant sympathy and understanding.

Yolaine turned to me. "Mama says it would have been better had you gone to Egypt. She says there are no pyramids in the Loire Valley."

I was grateful for a small shot of humor, however ironic. The grande dame and I looked at each other. Her eyes were misty and there was no mistaking the worried thoughts etched in the creases that lined her forehead. "*Au revoir et bon voyage, Richard,*" she said at last, and, despite her misgivings, I felt she meant it.

The intrigues and confrontations of the week past had left me emotionally whipped; but on the plane to the United

States, with the soft hum of the jets calming my nerves, with the vodka and a touch of cocaine mixing themselves up into a gentle euphoria in my brain, and with my woman beside me, I thought my way back over the events of the last two days at Teildras.

I knew that Le Comte was far from won over, but I felt that good progress had been made. For that matter, I was sure that even if he was outraged by the circumstances of my affair with his daughter, and no doubt truly concerned about the blunt questions he'd put to me, he had also been sizing me up in a different dimension altogether. Was it conceivable that this crazy American might actually be able to bring some help to his noble but debt-ridden family?

The family had a title, a heritage, and a magnificent piece of property, but no money. Yolaine's parents were getting old, and the hotel operation was barely keeping above water. What would happen to Teildras? I had not a little expertise in property development; as a consultant, I'd done the financial feasibility and marketing analyses for some big resort development projects. Perhaps I could do something for the family and my own account as well.

I'd learned enough about the French to know that, however intense their apparent preoccupation with matters of history, philosophy, and the spirit of life, their thoughts where personal relationships were concerned — whether friendship, casual social encounters, or family involvements — were seldom innocent of economic self-interest. The French were masters of the hidden agenda, and it usually involved money. Maybe Le Comte didn't like the lack of protocol in my relationship with his daughter, and maybe he looked askance at my unblooded pedigree; but if I came to the table with a way for the family to get out of its financial predicament, and ensure Teildras's survival for future generations of de Bernards, my blemishes would disappear as if by magic. I was sure of it.

So what if I didn't have any money? The family didn't know that; indeed, they had to believe the contrary. And I *did* have what was really needed — a lot of talent and usable contacts and the noblest of intentions. If I could get some kind of handle on the property, I could raise money and do wonderful things with the place. I'd turn it into a gold mine, become a hero to the family, get rich myself in the process, and give Yolaine the life she deserved. It would be a good idea for everybody.

The idea was so beautiful and, I was sure, so *doable*, that I decided to celebrate with a high-risk toot of cocaine. To hell with the bathroom. Yolaine's head had dropped over against my shoulder, but she was in such a deep sleep that I could manage it without disturbing her. As for the rest of the passengers, I'd take my chances. Cupping the vial out of sight between my knees, I dipped the spoon in, faked a coughing fit, took a quick snort up one nostril, and then repeated the routine. The rush was wonderful, Yolaine barely stirred, and I felt on top of life.

I took a big drink of vodka and pondered the events of the last two weeks. Despite four months of the best psychotherapy following my separation from Arlene, I had long since concluded that I could never truly love a woman — not in the *emotionally correct* way that the experts preached. But now, the cynicism that had taken a lifetime to create had been dispelled in the space of a couple of weeks, and I thought I had discovered the joy of just that kind of love.

Despite the affectionate efforts of my parents and siblings to identify and exorcise the demons that had somehow spiritually separated me from them, I had felt a foreigner in my own family all my life. Now, Yolaine had brought me a *glorious* family, in whose tradition and spirit I thought I could find a home.

I'd been in France only a short time, but I was leaving

the country with treasure. Yolaine was the crown jewel, but she wasn't all of it.

"Always remember who you are, Richard," my parents used to exhort me. I was never allowed to forget I was a son of pioneers and saints. The trouble was that, to me, our life had seemed thin and flat, as though even our love ran steady but shallow, without the passions of high mountains and deep valleys. Much of my youth had been spent in explorations outside my heritage — out beyond that flat desert of unleavened righteousness.

While still a boy, I had glimpsed a world in which the music was fuller, the clothes richer, the surfaces more rounded, the brains more complicated, the gods more devious. It was a voluptuous world, far removed from the arid, austere desert of noble struggle and narrow religious purpose that had infused my family with generations of righteousness and rectitude, but had emptied it of worldly visions and dulled the appetite for mortal feasts.

The unspoken purpose of my life had been to escape from the memories of the flat, arid world of my childhood and to come to fruition in the textured, voluptuous one. And, by God, it seemed at last to be happening. My beautiful French woman. Le Comte *et* La Comtesse, and generations of certified aristocracy. Fine wines and ancient tapestries. And Teildras itself, a four-century-old monument to heritage and position and place. Everything was coming together for me, and it all felt civilized, wonderful, and so absolutely *right*.

5
Miles to Travel . . .

T HE eight days with Yolaine in Washington and New
York were a whirlwind of sweet living. The weather
that early July was unseasonably wonderful for Washington — hot, but without the summer humidity that normally turned the town into a huge sweaty steambath. Every
inch of our suite at the Madison, with its subtle mix of
Federal and French decor, announced luxury and good
taste. Our room-service breakfasts were served punctually
on spotless linens. When our evenings on the town were
done, we'd return to find our nightly bottle of champagne
waiting in a gleaming bucket, and our small gold box of
chocolates on the table beside our turned-down bed.

I telephoned Ron, my former partner in San Francisco,
who had opened his own consulting firm in Washington,
and he and his wife, Christine, joined us for a lavish spread
of crab, oysters, caviar, and champagne in our suite, followed by dinner at Jacqueline's. I was glad to pay for it;
Ron was giving me some help on some lobbying, and I
could bill my client for expense reimbursement.

My first morning in town I went up to Capitol Hill to
see my friend Congressman X and pick up some cocaine.
All he had been able to produce was three grams; it wasn't
enough to meet the needs of the weeks ahead, but it was

a start. We'd had a chance to chat a little and have a few toots behind the locked door of his office in the Longworth Building; but he'd had to rush off to the floor of the House to vote, and I was looking forward to having him join us for dinner. I thought Yolaine would enjoy meeting a congressman and would be impressed.

Congressman X always wore his big Irish heart on his face, and that night it didn't look good. He and his wife were at each other most of the evening. Mrs. X took me off to the side and whispered that he was developing a serious cocaine problem. According to her husband, it was she who had the problem. "I think she's really becoming an addict," he told me as we sneaked a couple of toots in the men's room of the restaurant. "It's starting to affect our marriage." He warned me not to let her know he had some coke — "She can't handle it." After dinner, when Mrs. X and I were sipping drinks in the living room of their Capitol Hill house, while Yolaine and X were talking in the kitchen, she slipped me about half a gram in a vial. "Here's a little present from me to you. Don't worry, I've got plenty more. But, for God's sake, don't tell him I've got any. I've got to get him off the stuff before he kills himself."

"Sure, not a word," I promised. "And while we're on the subject, be sure that neither you nor he even *mentions* the subject to Yolaine; that's a pleasure she doesn't indulge in."

But even in a funk, Congressman X was always entertaining. So what if he had taken to eating like a slob, so what if his clothes were even more disheveled than usual and his unshaved face was puffy and gray? Despite a new testiness, he still had funny stories to tell and a few brilliant political insights to toss into the air. And I had seen a lot of spouses, during periods when they weren't getting along, lie about their cocaine use and hide their private stashes from each other.

Yolaine had not enjoyed herself. Back at the hotel, she said she thought the congressman a vulgar bore. I could only agree. It was true that his speech, always liberally sprinkled with colorful obscenities, had, with his appearance, sunk to a new level of seediness. I promised her the next night's festivities would be more refined.

I had lined up another friend from Congress for dinner at La Bagatelle. Mel had introduced me to Congressman Y a decade earlier, when Y was still at work making his millions as the head of his family-owned business. With his wealth secured, he had sold the business and taken off on a political career as one of California's foremost professional bleeding hearts. Lanky, handsome, and rich — and possessed of a blustering social conscience that could never stop announcing itself — Congressman Y was all noblesse oblige and easy charm.

He had gotten rid of his wife about the same time that Mel's, Michael's, and my marriages had dissolved. It must have been something in the air that year. Nearly fifty, he walked into La Bagatelle with a stunning nineteen-year-old brunette on his arm — a member of his "staff," he explained with a smile. As autumn-spring romances go, I thought I'd made an impressive move; but Y had beaten me in the age spread by about six years. I had long since learned that easy access to the favors of nubile beauties was a principal, if not widely publicized, congressional perquisite. "Power," as Henry Kissinger was reported to have told George Schultz when the latter asked him at a Georgetown party about his frequent appearances in the company of starlets, "is the world's greatest aphrodisiac."

Congressman Y performed wonderfully and relished every minute. His interminable but interesting political pontifications entertained Yolaine, and her studiously rapt attention fed his ever-hungry ego. We talked about France; Y said he was going there the next summer, and Yolaine advised him about good restaurants and chic beaches.

"Maybe we could all meet in Paris; how about lunch at La Brasserie Lipp?" I reminisced about old times in San Francisco and fondly gossiped about Mel and Michael and the rest of the gang. When I mentioned having had dinner with Congressman X, Congressman Y shook his head. "X has been acting odd and neglecting his work. I sure hope he's not going off the deep end with that stuff," he said very solemnly.

The evening was everything I'd hoped for. Yolaine got caught up in all the sophisticated political talk and was fascinated by our insiders' gossip about world events and shining people. In other circumstances, I might have been jealous of the attention she gave Congressman Y. But I had primed her to be especially attentive to him. I was doing a lot of business in Washington, Y was getting some seniority in Congress, and the time would come when I'd want his help. I had counted on Yolaine's charm as a subtle new weapon in my never-ending campaign of congressional ingratiation. Her evening's performance included some expert flirtation that I thought surpassed her assigned duties with a bit too much enthusiasm — but it was clear that she would be a great asset to me in both business and society, which, after all, came down to much the same thing.

Congressman Y said good-night and took his luscious teenager off to wherever congressmen take such friends at midnight before a big day of voting on the future of mankind, and Yolaine and I went to the street to find a taxi to take us to Blues Alley in Georgetown to hear some jazz. At the curb, Yolaine said, "Richard, tell me something. You're spending a fortune. You pay for everybody's dinners every night. Why don't any of your friends here pay for anything?"

For a woman from a culture where gracious avoidance of picking up a check had become an art form, it was a natural question, so I explained to her America's contribution to civilized living — the creative expense account. "It's important when dealing with government officials," I said, "and particularly so with congressmen. These people deliver millions of federal dollars to my clients, and all it costs the clients is my fees, some campaign contributions that I make in my own name and then get reimbursed for by loading the amounts into my invoices for fees, and a few high-priced dinners for our benefactors. My reimbursed expenses look awfully big each year, but they're nothing compared to the millions that come back in return. Besides, part of congressmen's unique charm is that they never pay for anything — not even the rich ones. Nobody really pays for any of this — including our suite at the Madison — except the taxpayers. And there are an awful lot of them to share the bill."

It was true that on occasion I had to fudge the vouchers with a little creative documentation. The dinner the night before hadn't been a problem; Mr. and Mrs. X were lawfully, if tenuously, wed, and a congressional spouse was as legitimate an expense for my broad-minded clients as was the great man she slept with. But I had to think a minute while writing my justification on the back of the La Bagatelle receipt. What would I call Miss Capitol Hill? I doubted that she could type or even make coffee. She'd spent the entire evening crossing and uncrossing her legs, turning one perfect profile and then the other toward me, laughing merrily at our jokes in all the wrong places, and her exquisite face going blank whenever a public policy issue had been discussed. But Congressman Y *had* introduced her as staff; so finally, I jotted down "congressman and staff," although I was reasonably certain that, whatever her job was, it seldom began before sundown.

If the Washington weather had been a pleasant surprise, New York's was close to paradise. With the mass exodus of midtown Manhattan's wives and children to their summer places in Connecticut and the Hamptons, the city's normally brutal pace had gone into its annual slowdown. Warmed by a gentle sun and invigorated by a crystal blue sky, we wandered the quiet streets, pretending to be serious shoppers at Tiffany's, doing a little modest but real shopping at Bendel's. I introduced Yolaine to the wonders of a New York hot dog and took her to Shakespeare in the Park and afternoon tea at the Plaza, where I dispatched the waiter to give the violinist ten dollars and a request for "I Love Paris."

With a phone call to the deputy director of the Port Authority, I managed to get a reservation at Windows on the World, the hottest spot in New York at the time.

"You'll get the best," my friend assured me. "After all, we own the goddamn building, don't we?"

And the best is what we got. Any friend of the Port Authority was a friend of the maître d'. As we sat at a window table in the southeast corner, looking down at the harbor from atop the huge slab that seemed to push against the very roof of the sky, Yolaine said simply, "Oh, my God," and I said, "It's really something, isn't it," and we both fell into an awed silence.

I remembered how lower Manhattan had looked when I first came to the town as a kid fresh out of law school. The first real skyscraper in the Wall Street area had been the Chase Manhattan Building and I remembered how, when I had been in town only a year, the firm had taken a couple of floors far up toward the top. God, I had been excited. My office, on the south side of that magnificent tower of steel and glass, looked out on the harbor, the way we were looking now, and I had thought I was sitting on top of the world. But after sitting up here, that old office would seem almost like street level. I wondered what sort of kid was sitting in my old office now, and what kind of view he had.

"See that string of lights over there?" I asked Yolaine.

"That's the Verrazano Bridge. They had just started building it when we left New York. It connects Brooklyn over there to the east with Staten Island — the cluster of lights you see way out in the harbor. That's where we lived."

In those days, with a little family and a peasant's income, Staten Island was the only decent place I could afford. Actually, it was kind of fun — full of hardworking Italians who lived in neat little middle-class houses, and went to their jobs and came back to their wives and kids every night at the same time. Besides, I knew it would be only a few years until I had my own fine brownstone on the Upper East Side.

Suddenly the past came back with an unsought clarity. The little park just two blocks from our flat where, on weekends, I played with Ursula. Lisa, just an infant then, parked in her pram and sucking a bottle under a shade tree. And the dining-room table I made out of an unfinished door slab that I stained to look like oak. I could still see the small brick duplex, the tiny flat with the pastel lavender walls, and, without realizing it, shook my head and smiled. "God, those were exciting times."

"More exciting than now, my love?" Yolaine's soft voice punctured my nostalgia, accusing me of unfaithfulness to the present.

"Oh God no, Yolaine, that wasn't what I meant. To be truthful, I was a lousy husband, although at the time I thought I was terrific. I loved my girls, but I neglected them. I didn't realize it then; it's just that, even when my work was finished, I always thought Manhattan more important than Staten Island; *that's* where the excitement was — in Manhattan, not at home. The truth is, except on weekends, I spent as little time as possible on Staten Island. Manhattan was where my work was, the dinners with clients, the art galleries, the elegant parties."

"But what about *now?*" Yolaine asked me. "Aren't you just as excited now? You've got money and a fine career;

and, from what I've seen of your friends, both in France and here, you ought to be positively drowning in excitement."

"Oh I am, I am," I enthused and meant it, but not without an ironic smile to myself over her unknowing but apt choice of a double-edged metaphor. "It's just that, however fantastic life is now, things are different when you're very young and, for the first time, really testing life.

"I don't want to run this nostalgia thing into the ground, sweetheart, but do you know what I got paid my first year in this town?" and I laughed at the thought of it. "Seven thousand and two hundred dollars a year; that's what everybody got the first year — even a young star like me — plus a thousand at Christmas. Do you know what a young lawyer straight out of school is getting on Wall Street now? Fifty thousand, that's what. It's obscene; no, actually, it's wonderful. Here's to them." And I raised my glass in a mock toast. "And to the demise of the Wall Street sweatshop."

I took a large gulp of my martini and with great heartiness said, "Well, enough of that; let's get on with the excitement of the present." I was dying for some coke. My small supply had dried up the night before and, with the week's frantic pace, fatigue and edginess were now doing battle with my charm for control of the evening's mood. Fortunately my friend Tony and his new girlfriend arrived and the moment was saved.

Tony was a former San Francisco colleague, who had been in New York for a couple of years working as the art director for a large ad agency. We always got together when I came to town, and it had been a happy convenience to have a lively old friend available who would drop everything to join me for dinner. Most important, he always could find me some coke at a moment's notice. His source was the best — his twenty-year-old art assistant who was the grandson and prospective heir of a former president of one of the world's largest banks.

Tonight Tony was his indomitable self — six feet two inches, a sturdy two-hundred-plus pounds, with red curly hair, a full red beard, and a rich basso voice that filled a room with jolly, carefully modulated thunder.

Tony and I gave each other big bear hugs, exchanged introductions, and I excused myself to make an "important phone call to a business associate in New Jersey." Without missing a beat, Tony picked up the cue and said that he would walk out with me since he had to visit the men's room. In the lobby by the elevators, he slipped me my plastic bag of coke and I slipped him his money. Tony had already stoked himself up — undoubtedly with some of the stuff he had just sold me — so he returned to the table while I made a pit stop.

I knew that, despite our close friendship, Tony had marked up the price of the coke; and both he and I knew, without discussing it, that I would pick up the tab for dinner. Tony dressed straight out of *Gentlemen's Quarterly* — once he'd shown up at a car race at Laguna Seca in ninety-degree weather wearing a full set of Harris tweeds and a hat, and carrying a birdwatcher's chair — and he lived every hour of his life first class. Consequently, despite his hefty earnings as one of the country's truly eminent graphic designers, he was always broke. However much he earned, he always spent more; most of it on indulgences of high taste — clothes, apartment furnishings and art, and appropriate cars. With the growth of his expensive coke appetite, neither his wardrobe nor life-style had suffered; all that changed was an increase in his long-standing operating deficit. None of his friends minded easing the strain or that he took a profit on the coke. He was a gentleman's gentleman, an outrageously gifted raconteur, and a warm friend.

Tony mentioned that his agency was planning to shoot

photographs for perfume ads on location in France, using a château, and that he might go over to supervise the project. Yolaine and I exchanged a meaningful glance. I hadn't told her of my plans for Teildras; they were still germinating in my mind. Despite our love, it still seemed too soon to disclose my hunger for the grand old house with its meadows and oak trees. Too soon a move might make her wonder. But that night, as quickly as I, she picked up on the possibility of getting Tony to shoot the photographs at Teildras.

Whatever the subject, Yolaine was always quick on the uptake — sometimes too much so for comfort — and I sensed that she was about to mount a charming hustle. I shook my head at her ever so slightly and shot her a little frown, and she got the message. She swallowed the unvented thought, but not without giving me a puzzled look that said, with a touch of pique, Why shouldn't I? It was a conversation I was glad to have squelched before it began. Whatever I was to bring to Teildras, from an invaluable piece of international publicity to a development plan worth millions, I wanted to be sure that Le Comte was unmistakably clear that it was indeed *I* who brought it. Yolaine was smart enough to be my partner in all things, and God knows I wanted it that way; but, at best, mixing the de Bernard family and business would be like walking through a minefield, and I wanted control of the journey from beginning to end.

We went down from the tower and got a cab for a short ride to the Village for some jazz. Tony and I kept ourselves high and amusing on coke, and he regaled Yolaine through the night with dirty jokes made elegant by the savoir faire of their telling, and with anecdotes of the good old days with Mel, Michael, and me, freely indulging his storyteller's license and inventing a few hilarities that never happened. Even sober, Tony was a delight; on coke, he was outrageous.

We got back to the Sherry-Netherland just after mid-night — early for us in those whirlwind days — and Yo-laine gave me my nightly massage with the body cream she had bought for me on our last day in Paris. I was exhausted and, for once, her expert, loving hands brought sleep instead of arousal, and we both lay unconscious until ten in the morning. A night of sleep instead of two A.M. champagne and passion was just what I needed in prep-aration for our last evening in town, for I had saved the best for last.

It had been about a decade since the Brokaws had left Los Angeles to plow the more fertile fields of national network television; but, despite the fact that I saw them only three or four times a year on my trips east, we had remained fast friends. Tom was hosting the "Today" show then, a way station between his White House correspon-dent assignment and his much-rumored ascent to the na-tional anchorman spot on the "Nightly News" when John Chancellor retired. And even though it was a weeknight, and Tom had to get up at four-thirty the next morning to get ready for the show, he and his wife, Meredith, had enthusiastically accepted my invitation to dinner to meet my probable future wife.

We all set off in Tom's limousine for a restaurant in the Village, where he had made reservations. The Tulip was an elegant but unpretentious place with first-rate food that, as Tom explained, had become a favorite of media people who wanted to be left alone. The significance of the menu's reasonable prices wasn't lost on me. After years of being entertained by the Brokaws in Washington and New York, I'd insisted that they would be my guests or we wouldn't go at all, and, ever-thoughtful, Tom had picked out a place more congenial to my wallet than to his. Despite all the years of flash, Tom sensed how it really was with me, living close to the margin.

It was a good evening, but not a great one. We talked

about some of the good times we'd had together — the week skiing at Tahoe with Arlene and me, the week together in Utah when, one night, Tom and I had trudged through the snow to a Park City bar to shoot some pool, hustled a couple of local toughs into a game, and with an incredible streak of luck for two really incompetent players, walked away with the pot, certain in our hearts that we were men marked for physical vengeance.

As we were waiting for coffee, Yolaine put on some lipstick and brushed her hair, and I said, "Sweetheart, I really wish you wouldn't do that at the table."

Yolaine suddenly looked mad — I'd given her that speech before without incident — and Meredith butted in with "Why shouldn't she? I always put on lipstick at the table; after all, Dick, we *are* living in the twentieth century."

"Well, lipstick maybe isn't so bad; but it really is quite tacky to brush hair all over everybody's plates."

Tom guffawed and said, "Some things never change. Yolaine, before you go much further, you really should know that, despite his pretenses of enlightenment, you're running around with one of the great sexists of our time," and then proceeded to recall — as I was certain he would — the time in a restaurant at Tahoe when, at dinner, I had put Arlene down for a dumb remark. I had done it in great good humor, but Arlene hadn't been amused. The Brokaws had never forgotten it, and the incident had become another staple of the lore of our long friendship that they loved to dredge up at every appropriate opportunity.

"See," Yolaine said, as if on the crest of a great triumph.

It was a small thing but I was getting edgy. I'd excused myself several times during dinner to call "my business associate in New Jersey," but for some reason the coke wasn't working right. Maybe I simply had done too much the past week. Or maybe it was because I was all alone in my pleasure. It was one of the few times when, out in a group, I hadn't had at least one companion in my secret.

193

And it definitely wasn't any fun to be surreptitiously snorting alone among a bunch of nonusers; not even a *single soul* to exchange knowing smiles with across the table in silent acknowledgment of our mutual euphoria. In fact, that night there *wasn't* any euphoria — I was a little more awake, maybe, but none of the usual rush, none of the surge of well-being.

I wished I could invite Tom back to the bathroom for a toot, but that would be taking too big a chance. In all of our heady times together, I'd never seen him alter his brain with anything stiffer than a few glasses of wine. Hell, he wasn't even smoking an occasional cigarette; he was jogging, looking incredibly fit, and acting altogether like the hero of a health spa commercial. I loved him mightily, but that night, without any good reason that came consciously to mind, I began to resent him just a little.

And I thought Tom's usual warmth had flagged as the evening had worn on. Maybe it was because he and Meredith had liked Arlene and felt uncomfortable. Maybe it was because they suspected the drug. And maybe I was simply the victim of a dose of coke paranoia.

If, for me, the night had seemed a little off the mark, for Yolaine it was a great delight. She adored the Brokaws and had found her first chauffeured limousine ride very much to her taste.

While we waited at JFK for her flight to Paris the next day, she said that she had loved New York, and had fallen in love with me even more in that wonderful place. "New York's even better than Washington," she said.

We spent a couple of hours together in the terminal sipping Bloody Marys and holding hands, unable to say much. She was on the verge of tears; my own pain at our parting grew with the minutes.

When they announced that her plane was ready for boarding, I took both her hands in mine. "Sweetheart, I promise you I'll come to France in August, and we'll make plans then. I love you."

"Write to me," she said.

"I will."

"And telephone me."

"I will."

"Promise me."

"I promise — with all my heart."

As she walked through the metal detector and down the corridor toward the gate, I felt the shock of sudden aloneness. After three short weeks, I felt as though we had been together all our lives, and already I needed her.

She had been right to insist on the trip; it had been wonderful. As always seemed to be the case in such matters, I had grossly underestimated the cost. But to hell with the cost; it had been a smart investment. Yolaine had experienced my life — well, at least the glittering surface of it, the important part — and, immersed in the splendors of two great cities, we had forged a closeness that I knew could never be breached by any intruding person or problem, however threatening. And, romance aside, the trip would have a practical payoff. She would return to her parents with tales of congressmen and artists, of media stars and limousines. There would be reports of fashionable restaurants and choice old wines; of wealth and dear friends and love, all of a piece. And the family would be impressed. And the marriage would be set with parental blessings. And the doors would swing open not only to love, but to opportunity as well.

Although my blood ran heavy with alcohol and drugs, and my mind was festering with Byzantine schemes, I had never seen my innocence so clearly; I felt as clean as a young boy.

An hour later, aboard the plane to San Francisco, as the stewardess helped me into my seat, nothing in the bright panorama of luxury and love that stretched across my reeling brain hinted that my future might end up a lonely one. I haven't seen the Brokaws since. And there are many other dear old friends who would find the path I was on too treacherous and would stay behind on firmer ground; I wouldn't have time for formal good-byes.

It was a relief when the plane reached cruising altitude and the seat belt sign went off. I hurried to the restroom and helped myself to the largest dose of cocaine I had ever had at one time, returned to my seat for some more gin, and settled down for the flight home. I had been gone a month, and my life had changed.

I missed Yolaine, but it was a joy to be back home. I knew we'd be reunited soon, and, in the meantime, all the elated gossip about our romance kept her image vividly alive, an almost palpable presence.

Lounging in the Sunday sun on Michael's deck, at dinner with James and Catherine in their renovated farmhouse, over fine port wine with Mel and Nina at a little French bistro, all the talk was of Richard's great adventure with the countess.

"Well, Richard," Michael said, "you've always really been an aristocrat at heart and you truly deserve a château of your own." And he added, with the affectionate irony of a multimillionaire who for years had been financing much of his poorer friend's fast-track life, "I just hope you'll remember your old buddies when we want to come and visit."

But I had a lot to do in the next six weeks before returning to Yolaine. First I had to pacify my clients. I had told the directors of the Golden Gate Bridge that I'd be gone only a couple of weeks, and I hadn't told the folks in Philadelphia that I was going at all. The former would be agitated — my negotiations with the federal government for many millions of dollars to put a deck on the bridge were at a critical juncture — and the latter would be mad as hell; they hadn't the slightest idea of their project's status, and I'd been unreachable for a month.

I would have to do some fast talking to justify good-sized invoices for the "work" I did on their behalf during Yolaine's and my stay in Washington. That was cash I had to get in my bank account immediately or I'd find myself in very deep water indeed, and my request for expedited payment might raise some skeptical eyebrows in light of my protracted holiday. And, even with that accomplished, there would be the need to invent enough "critical" new work to bill my clients another ten thousand dollars, and get paid for it before my departure at the end of August.

It might be a dicey business, but my clients still thought me a unique sort of genius at extracting big money from the feds, they needed me badly, and I would convince them of the need to quickly infuse some nourishment into my anemic cash flow. With a lot of charm, and some dollops of the self-deprecating humor that never failed to ingratiate — "Oh, come on, you know how it is; haircuts cost a fortune these days, and the alimony's killing me; show a little understanding for the idle poor" — I'd always managed to cajole my clients' controllers into accelerating payment, and this time would be no different. With my expenditures nearly always running ahead of my income now, the plea had become a practiced routine.

I drove to the bank to visit my loan officer. As anticipated, he had paid the several thousand dollars of over-drafts that had come in from the trip so far, but he was unusually testy.

"Look, you've really got to start reducing some of this debt," Frank said. "I've worked with you on your cash flow problems, and I'm going to continue to work with you, but you've got to start performing."

"What's the big deal?" I asked. "You've carried a lot more of my debt than this in the past; you know I'm eventually good for it."

"*You* know you're good for it, and *I* know you're good for it; but the bank examiner doesn't know that. The examiner's due in here any day now; he's going to make us categorize this fistful of overdrafts as loans; and, unless there's some performance, he's going to classify the whole goddamn mess a bad debt. *That's* what the 'big deal' is.

"I can't have that happen, Dick; I just can't. You and a few other people have got me in a helluva bind. I spend half my time trying to keep the loan files of you special customers reasonably clean. But it's damn tough. I know that, if I come down hard on you, you'll go bitching to Mel, and he'll summon me across town to his office and yell his favorite speech at me. You know, the bullshit about banking being a *people*-oriented business and how I've got to be more sensitive and understanding toward the bank's loyal old, highly favored, customers. Which, of course, means you and his other buddies. And, getting the message, I'll lay off you; and then get more shit from my own boss about my *again* having the worst goddamn bad loan record in the bank."

"Hell, Frank, I didn't know I was giving you such a problem; I keep forgetting about the bank examiner," I said. "I'll tell you what I'll do. There's no way I can pay down any of the principal on the loan now. But what if I bring the interest current and pay off the overdrafts in the first couple of weeks in August? Will that help?"

"Do I have a choice?" he said.

"No. But one other thing, Frank. I'm really surprised that you think I'd use leverage with Mel to get you to give me special treatment. I've been working with you personally for several years now, and never once have I used my friendship with him to get you to approve a loan."

Strictly speaking, that was true, but of course Frank

was aware that I consulted Mel from time to time when I was nervous about a potential problem at the bank and thought it wise to protect myself. It was nice to have a close friend who was not only a client, but also a major stockholder and the biggest customer of my bank. Indeed, among Mel's many influences, his power at the bank was perhaps the most important; and he freely used it on his close friends' behalf. A word from Mel could quickly change a bank officer's threats regarding a delinquent loan into an attitude of benign tolerance. Just that morning, in fact, I had stopped by Mel's office near Union Square for a few minutes on my way to see Frank. My couple of minutes' visit had stretched into an hour after I tipped a goodly mound of cocaine out on a magazine on top of his big oak desk. By the time we were through, we'd finished off a gram. At the going price in those days, that represented a hundred and ten dollars, but I didn't mind. Mel was always a kick to spend time with, and it had been a damn good investment in my overall liquidity.

As I rose to go, Mel said, "Hey, Richard, wait a minute. You know your consulting contract with my company" — a few months earlier he had hired me to lobby some legislation in Washington for some of his foreign clients — "how much is that for? Fifty thousand, isn't it? Look, if you're really in bad financial shape, let's amend the contract. You're worth a hell of a lot more than that. When you get back from France, give me a proposal revising it up to seventy-five grand."

The windfall came like a gift from heaven, and I had thanked him warmly. "Oh, hell, it's not that big a deal," he said. "Besides, I know you'll earn it." And then, almost as an afterthought, he had dropped the other shoe. "Oh, and Richard, as I told you, I'm in a temporary bind myself. After you get a couple of invoices paid, it would be great if you could loan me ten of it."

After my initial elation I felt discomfiture. Was he talking loan, or was he talking kickback? I'd mumbled that that was something we could talk about when the time came, thanked him again, and said good-bye.

After leaving Mel's office, I walked up Broadway for lunch alone at Enrico's. It was one of those days that make you think you'd have to be crazy to want to live anyplace but San Francisco. The fog had burned off, the breeze was soft, and the sky was evened out in a pristine blue, without even the wisp of a vapor trail to scar its face.

I settled in at an outside table, over a spinach crêpe and a glass of white wine. The street was alive with its usual motley midday crowd. Executives, lawyers, and their girlfriends hurrying to lunch at Vanessi's; barkers trying to hustle strolling tourists into seedy topless joints; the Thunderbird winos and glue-sniffers come down from their North Beach hangouts to warm their hangovers in the sun. I watched a couple of long-legged brunettes wearing hip huggers and summer halters, and looking very much in love, walk up toward Columbus and then cross Broadway, en route no doubt to City Lights, where they would browse through Ferlinghetti's fabulous gold mine of esoteric literature until they found just the right piece of arty pornography with which to while away a lazy summer afternoon.

It felt good to be back in my gentle, beautiful, yeasty town again, and good to be in love there, even though my love was a continent and an ocean away. I had never — not in my whole life — felt so secure. There was only one small cloud on my happiness: Mel's proposition. God knows, I needed the fifteen thousand I would net after "loaning" him the money he wanted. But I'd never done anything like that in my life. Sure, I had cut some corners in business, but nothing that wasn't common practice among basically honest, yet sophisticated, businessmen. I'd become adept at using client expense accounts to maximize my own enjoyments — everybody with any brains did that — but even there, I was fairly scrupulous about making sure that my client was getting *some* benefit, however indirect, from the expenditures. And, however much my clients had paid me, I'd always prided myself in giving real value back.

This was something else altogether. Would it really be a loan, or was it a dressed-up embezzlement? I knew that paying kickbacks to get business was common practice with a lot of people, but it just wasn't my style. I still had a conscience left.

I thought about Mel's slide the last few years, and felt sorry for him. He was still the bon vivant to the hilt, and a warm and caring friend. But his erosion had been steady and ugly. Nina's frequent black eyes and swollen nose. The all-night orgies of pot, booze, coke, and Quaaludes, complete with easy seduction of friends' drug-besotted girlfriends. The couple's incessant public fights that embarrassed their friends and left maître d's stunned in angry helplessness. And now it was to be embezzlement.

I knew that coke was a large part of their problem, and I was glad that, despite my love of the stuff, I'd been able to control my use of it. While it badly distorted some people's personalities and ruined their judgment, others seemed able to handle it nicely, energized and made better by its power rush. I was glad I'd turned out to be one of the lucky ones.

Besides, my use was moderate as seriously engaged coke users go. Maybe twelve thousand dollars' worth in the last year, I figured. But Mel — my God, he had to be spending two to three times that, especially with all the stuff he was giving away to attract the company of the rock musicians he and Nina had become fascinated with, not to mention his continued, although recently diminished, generosity with his old friends. And that was on top of what he was paying to put Nina's children through California's most exclusive private schools. On top of the luxury trips to

Acapulco, the imported luxury cars, and the hundred-dollar bottles of wine. Even with enormous expenditures for coke, Mel wasn't about to compromise his life-style, and I was sure that the extra load of the drug purchases was the straw that was going to break his back — unless he could pick up some more income. But kickbacks from consultants? I wasn't prepared for the proposition and it depressed me. I wondered how many others he was trying to do that kind of business with. I didn't want to go along with it; that was a compromise I wasn't yet prepared to make.

Well, it was a decision I could postpone for a couple of months. Maybe Mel would be in better shape by then, and I could get the extra money on my contract without the problem. I gulped the rest of my wine and, for the time being, put the matter out of my mind.

July and August passed quickly, taken up with days of intense work to generate cash, and nights of intense play with a new friend to fill the empty hours when neither Mel, Michael, nor James was available. I had promised myself to be faithful to Yolaine, although neither of us had demanded or given such a pledge. I simply wanted to — it was a matter of proof of character. So I had a lot of time to get to know Greg.

In my experience, Greg was a different breed of drug dealer. After George finished law school, and he and his wife quit dealing coke, a carpenter friend had introduced me to Greg. George and Joanne had a lot of class and they had been largely society dealers; the preponderance of Greg's business was with less rarefied types. I had bought coke from Greg a number of times before I had left for France, and — although we were from far different worlds — we liked each other. He was a bartender at a hip wood-and-glass place filled with hanging ferns in Sausalito. In what was left of 1979, I spent much of my spare time with Greg there. Although credit transactions were out of favor in the drug world, Greg put me on the cuff with much goodwill. He not only liked me; he trusted the Montgomery Street cut of my suits. I had just returned from a jaunt in France and was hardly the kind of customer that would turn out to be a deadbeat.

Greg's bar was only a five-minute drive from my house and a great convenience, although its crowd wasn't quite what I was used to. There were, among the regulars, a number of three-piece-suit types — hotshot young stock-brokers and junior executives on their way up, who took the ferry from the city to Marin and stopped by the bar for a couple of drinks, and maybe to arrange a tryst with one of the waitresses or barflies, before going on home to the wife and kids.

Apart from them, the crowd was all downhill. Sausalito is a boat town, and the bar was where the boat people — or those who styled themselves as such — hung out. Not the kind who docked their boats at the St. Francis Yacht Club in San Francisco, or up in Tiburon, with the sleek, pricey equipment; but the kind whose boats were marginal at best, and the kind who had no boats at all. Almost *everybody* in the bar crowd — carpenters, part-time bartenders, and other odd-jobbers — was, it seemed, a former America's Cup crew member. And all of them were always just having a few drinks before joining the crew of some boat that they were about to sail for so-and-so down to San Pedro, or on the Trans-Pac race to Hawaii. But the "few drinks" stretched into weeks and months. And they all had some big potential business deal simmering that would soon come to a boil and bring the justly deserved wealth they had once had before their streak of bad luck. Everybody at Greg's bar, it seemed, had either been something and somebody, or was just about to become something and somebody. But it happened that nobody was anything or anybody at just that precise, unfortunate moment.

The one thing that nearly everybody at the bar had in common was their cocaine hunger. If you happened into the place and weren't looking for coke, you obviously were lost. While the Sausalito hills were an elegant bedroom community for prosperous professionals and business people who worked in the city, the commercial center of the once-charming fishing village had become a tourist trap for strangers and, for the downtown locals, a place of waiting. Waiting for boats, for the "big deal," for drugs and getting laid. The boats seldom showed up and the big deals never did; but the drugs and quick sex were plentiful. Sausalito was Marin's drug depot, Greg's bar was the main place, and Greg was the Main Man.

I liked the times at Greg's bar. I was a newcomer but was good at adapting, and the regulars and I soon were easy drinking buddies. Why not? I was buying. It was a good change of pace. I had spent my recent years trying to keep up with my much richer friends; among this bunch of broke bullshitters, I was an aristocrat in both money and manner, but no snob, and we enjoyed each other. Greg would serve me my first drink and look at me solemnly and ask, "Are you feeling in need?" and I would say, "Oh yes, I'm feeling very much in need," and he would say, "Here's a fresh napkin for your glass," and I would surreptitiously remove from the fold of the napkin a paper bindle containing a gram of coke, employing a slickness of hand that neatly concealed the transaction and gave me a rush of high-risk excitement. The undercover narcotics agents who were said to frequent the bar had been foiled again — and right before their very eyes. And Greg nonchalantly would reach into the canvas shoulder bag that he stowed behind the bar, pull out the stack of yellow, three-by-five file cards, flip through them until he found the one with my name on it, and, moistening the lead point of his pencil on the tip of his tongue, would add another hash mark to the ledger. With me, Greg was generous with his credit and ruthless in his record-keeping; and his soiled canvas bag was his portable office.

When Greg wasn't working the bar, I spent a lot of time in his house. En route, we would drive very slowly up Bridgeway to ensure that Sausalito's police wouldn't have an excuse to stop us and search Greg and the car on some pretext. It was common knowledge that Greg was one of the biggest dealers in the county, and he assumed that his ten-year-old Mercedes convertible was number one on every cop's prime target list.

We were an oddly matched couple cruising the street with the top down — he in the sheepskin jacket and dark brown cowboy hat that were the costume of choice among Sausalito's supercool, compulsively macho studs, and I in my summer pinstripes and Hermès silk tie. Greg was the Marlboro Man incarnate, and indeed that was his official cigarette; I was the refined establishment fellow from uptown, who puffed his effetely mentholated Salem Light. But what we lacked in common imagery we made up for in our shared passion for the drugs he purveyed; and in the fantasies and far-out humor we could share when smoking and snorting. Pot and coke made all of us devotees the same in spirit if not in circumstances, breaking down barriers of class, time, and place, and creating a new community of understanding.

From my observations, I had thought that Greg did a lot of business at the bar. As August unfolded, and I increasingly became a semipermanent fixture at his nightly soirees, I was amazed to discover that he did ten times that amount at home, generally between seven in the evening and three in the morning — except when the mood was exceptionally good and the favored few were invited to stay until dawn.

The clientele was eclectic. Greg prided himself on having been married five times and, with a logic uniquely his own, bragged that all the marriages had been "successful" because the women all still loved him — and he, them — and he still helped them with their problems. Two of them who lived in the area were in the house almost nightly. From what I could see, Greg "helped" them mainly by keeping them in coke and, with everybody high as a kite, giving them philosophical advice on how to manage their lives with their various boyfriends.

One of the ex-wives, a big blonde who once had been beautiful but was now tending toward trussed-up sagginess and a storm-weathered face that had seen it all, was living with a young lawyer who, despite his heavy coke habit, was angling politically for a judgeship. The other was a willowy brunette who lived with a local woodworking artisan who also was an addict of every drug on the street; his rich mother in the East sent him a reasonable allowance every week, but it never was enough for the drugs that had turned his eye sockets hollow. Whenever he got too far in hock and Greg cut off his coke supply, either Greg's ex-wife would show up alone to plead on his behalf, or the boyfriend would show up himself with a beautiful inlaid table he had made, or some other elegant piece of work, and he and Greg would make a trade.

Neither of Greg's ex-wives seemed to mind his live-in girlfriend, nor she them. Jeanette was a blond, not-very-smart stewardess, and when she was flying — and sometimes when she wasn't — Greg would help his ex-wives, as well as the assortment of cocktail waitresses and other men's wives who were his regular guests, "solve their problems" not only with coke and trenchant advice, but by bedding them.

All of the women had three things in common — washed-out faces permanently fixed in blankness, not quite enough money to support their habits, and Greg's coke.

And to have Greg's coke in common was to have Greg in common.

He would often wax eloquent on the despicable character of men who got their sex by exploiting "coke whores." A coke whore wasn't a hooker in the usual sense; she could be a wife, a girlfriend, a corporate executive — any woman who was easier if you had some coke. He didn't see himself that way at all. He was an eminent philosopher-businessman conducting soirees and solving people's problems. And he truly believed that the women loved him as he loved all people. His coke, he kidded himself with total persuasion, was wholly incidental to their passion and their solicitation of his "wisdom."

I could understand Greg's unshakable belief in his attractiveness to women. Although he was forty-six and starting to show the ravages of the drugs, he was still healthy and vigorous in those days, and he cut a striking figure. With a full head of curly brown hair only beginning to go gray and a rugged, open face that could only be called handsome, he had not yet begun to surrender to the incipient softness that eventually transforms many overly handsome men into strangely effete, decadent caricatures of their younger selves.

He was actually deeply sensitive, and often he favored not only his women, but also his men friends with the poetry he composed late at night on a yellow pad while sitting in his hot tub, then painstakingly copied onto parchment in a fine calligraphy. It was poetry of love and birth and death and friendship, often disjointed by too many drugs, but always in meter and freighted with caring insights.

He claimed to have once been a lawyer, though I doubted that he had ever been admitted to the bar. Nor did I believe that he had once been the president of a hot venture capital company in Chicago that sold sophisticated medical management systems, or that, before his luck had run bad with his bankrupted company, he had been a prized crew member on the country's elite racing yachts out of Newport and Long Island. But I was wrong on the latter two counts, as I would learn a long time later when, as partners of a sort, we would travel to Chicago and New York together, and I would discover that he had indeed been a promising young businessman, as well as a yachtsman of note. He wasn't going to be a coke dealer the rest of his life, he assured me. "This is just a temporary thing to keep me in some money until I can get myself back in the mainstream."

Greg obviously had had a sharp mind, until it got saturated with drugs. And even now, his ideas showed flashes of brilliance, before they crescendoed into disarray, as they always did, with too many sentences piled endlessly on top of each other in an inverted pyramid made top-heavy by the flashy but increasingly discursive ramblings of pot and coke. I felt for Greg — for his sensitivity, for his caring, and for the possibilities he had once had before the drugs had gotten at his core. I liked him a lot. And I was glad for myself. Glad that I didn't have Greg's problem. Glad that I had my drug use under control; and that I had a verifiable past, an honorable present, and a future of unlimited opportunity — a life of reality instead of pathetic illusion.

Tommy the Thief invariably dropped in around midnight. "Hi, Tommy the Thief," people would say, "how's it going?" He was the top man at his profession in Marin County. Whatever you wanted at a half to two-thirds off the retail price, Tommy the Thief could get for you. His specialty was top-of-the-line electronic gear — stereos, televisions, VCRs, video cameras. Some of the stuff obviously had been lifted from homes, but a lot of it came in unopened shipping boxes, procured from longshoreman thieves on the San Francisco docks.

About five feet four inches of nothing but skin and

bones, and reeking of days of stale sweat, Tommy the Thief looked and acted like a weasel. He was a hard-core addict who liked to mix up a batch of his heroin with some of Greg's coke and mainline it into a vein. He'd come bursting into Greg's house with an ashen face shining with sweat and a clammy hand that he insisted on shaking with everybody, while urgently muttering, "Where's Greg, where's Greg? Got to see about Greg. Got some major business with Greg," in a tone that sounded as if he was about to propose a sale and lease-back of the TransAmerica Building.

And Greg would drop whatever he was doing and shepherd Tommy into a tiny back office, and Tommy the Thief would come out a few minutes later and lock himself in the bathroom for twenty minutes, after which he'd emerge calmed down and looking better, having tied off a vein with his little rubber rope and shot himself up with that night's salvation.

We all hated Tommy the Thief because he was ugly and obnoxious and had no class, but most of all because he was a heroin addict and represented the sordid underside of the drug world. His mere presence threatened the smug complacency with which we indulged our pleasure. In Tommy the Thief, there was no way I could see even a pale image of myself.

As summer's end approached, I was aware that my life had taken an odd turn; I was traveling on two tracks. I was still working hard most days, meeting with my clients, making presentations to boards of directors, telephoning congressmen, and taking a couple of quick flights to Washington to expedite my clients' interests. And half of my social life continued to complement my professional one. There were the theater and the summer symphony with James and Catherine, and the after-theater suppers in Trader Vic's Captain's Cabin. And the dinners with Michael and Alice — French cuisine at the little bistro, and high Italian at Garimonti's. And tennis at the Belvedere Club, where I kept up my tan.

It wasn't that the nights at Greg's, which seemed to grow longer as the summer wore on, were evil departures from an otherwise saintly existence. Except when I went out with James and Catherine, cocaine was ubiquitous in both of my worlds. And it was *good* in both places. The pleasures were just *different* at Greg's place. There was a lot more coke, for one thing. And you could do it all night long, without sneaking off to restaurant bathrooms between courses. And there wasn't the need to be onstage all the time, preening and pontificating for the approving attention of society columnists and headwaiters. At Greg's tiny house, tucked away in a grove of trees against the side of a hill, you were in a private place devoted exclusively to the serious business at hand, a business that, in the city's elite restaurants and in my other friends' elegant parlors, was only a hobby, albeit a much-loved one. Among Greg's other guests, I had no need to strain to impress; I was self-evidently a cut above them.

It wasn't that I was about to abandon the world of glitter, glamour, and establishment achievement, and hook myself up in a serious way with the Sausalito waterfront crowd. Far from it. I still had my ambitions and plans intact. But I found Greg's crowd incredibly relaxing. Best of all, I could get as much coke as I wanted with as much credit as I needed, and, given my plans for the future, the credit was important.

A couple of days before I was to return to France, I spent the whole night at Greg's. It was around four in the morning, and most of the patrons had said their goodnights. The exceptions were a talented odd-jobber who had installed an electronically controlled security door in Greg's office in return for some coke, one of the ex-wives, and Al the lawyer, the only Montgomery Street type besides me who did regular business with Greg. Al was alseep on the big sofa after a night of heavy tooting while conferring with Greg and me about his mounting financial crisis and the various fanciful schemes he had concocted for getting out of it. And the ex-wife and the odd-jobber had long since crashed in a sleeping bag on the floor.

Greg and Jeanette and I were too revved up to sleep, and we soaked ourselves in the hot tub out on the deck, smoking pot, taking an occasional snort, drinking wine, looking at the stars, and contemplating the goodness of life.

"Dick, have you ever tried any amyl?" he asked.

I told him that I hadn't, but that I knew about it and wouldn't mind finding out what was so exciting about it. Amyl nitrate was a cardiac stimulant manufactured for emergency use by heart patients. Gays were said to have been the first to have discovered the rush of ecstasy that a whiff of it could bring if perfectly timed a couple of seconds before orgasm; and, as word of its magic had spread, amyl had become a favorite among those folks who, regardless of sexual orientation, searched endlessly for the elusive, perfect drug that would transform mere sex into a cosmic explosion.

"Well, now's a perfect time for you to try a shot," Greg said, as he dried his hands on a towel on the redwood shelf at the side of the tub, and reached for the ever-present canvas bag in which he surely must have carried a drug to pacify every need and taste, with only heroin, apparently, excepted from the exotic inventory.

"Great," I said, "but unfortunately there's no woman around to participate in my baptism." And I tossed Jeanette a look of mock apology and said, "No offense intended, dear."

"Oh, shit, Richard, it's great with balling, that's true," Greg said. "But that's not its only happy use. When you're mellowed out on good pot and wine, a jolt or two of amyl's the greatest — sex or no sex."

He took a Vick's inhaler out of the bag and a tiny glass ampul wrapped in fabric mesh, removed the inhaler's nosepiece from its cylinder, threw away the menthol cartridge, sharply cracked the ampul open with his two thumbnails, quickly dropped it into the cylinder, and put his thumb over the hole of the nosepiece before the fumes could escape. He waded across the big wood tub to where I sat in steaming-hot water up to my armpits. "Here, Dick, have a couple of hits of paradise," he said, with the warm urgency of a friend, and stuck the inhaler into each of my nostrils while he held the other one closed with his thumb, and I twice sniffed the stuff up deep into my sinuses.

In an instant, as my heart raced and a burning heat rushed into my head and seared my face with a tingling flush, and a wave of nausea swept over my body, I was enveloped in fear; it was a toss-up which would kill me — a heart burst open by a massive coronary, or the stroke that would surely shatter my brain. But then, the nausea passed and with it the fear, as the throbbing in my head settled down into a marvelous buzz; and the brain that I had been sure would explode instead took up a wild and wonderful dance. Deep in the water, I felt my penis enlarge, its head as responsive as the most sensitive thermostat to the wet, luxurious heat.

Greg and Jeanette had each had their hits and we looked into each other's sweating faces, now beet-red from the flush of a million capillaries enlarged and engorged with rushing blood. We laughed hilariously. And then we simply gazed at each other with swimming eyes and said, "Oh, wow!"

Yolaine had insisted that the bulk of my return trip to France not be spent at Teildras among the family, but alone with her, swimming in the Mediterranean, sunbathing on white sands, and dancing the nights away in far-removed places. She had always loved Saint-Tropez and wanted us to go there, so that's what we did the last week of August. She had suggested that we stay at Biblos, the luxurious white hotel, terraced on a hill in the middle of town, that was favored by the rich and famous. But there was no way I could afford it and I told her so. By then our relationship was secure enough that I felt at ease finally telling her that, despite appearances, there were some limits to my spending. It was hardly the whole truth, just enough to impose some constraints without sounding an alarm that might give rise to second thoughts. And I said it with an offhanded humor that signaled nothing more ominous to my sweetheart than that she was in love with a man who, notwithstanding his generous spirit, was prudent in the management of his affairs.

So Yolaine had consulted with her friends and located a wonderful little cluster of stucco cottages with tile roofs out on the peninsula, about halfway between the town and the beach. And despite the fact that it was owned by Belgians and all the other patrons were Belgians — Yolaine airily dismissed *les Belges* as poor French cousins who spoke the language badly, cooked badly, dressed badly, were often fat and always pretentious, and had no class — we had a delightful time there, loving each other through the soft summer nights and taking our coffee by the pool, before our jaunts to town or beach.

One afternoon we spent hours watching the local old men in their berets play at *la boule* in the park that stretched down the center of an avenue crowded with tourists. It was a game of incredibly slow motion. The grapefruit-sized steel balls barely moved down the dirt alley, seeming always on the verge of running out of steam, yet rolling on and on and on, until they approached that precise spot where the callused hands that had launched their journeys had willed them to stop. For Yolaine and me, it was a wonderful hour of respite in simplicity, and we whispered about how fine it would be to have a second house one

213

day in the south of France. Maybe a great old stone house that we could remodel in the hills above Aix, where we could read and listen to music and hike in the hills and ride horses. And on Saturday afternoons I would go down to the village and play *la boule*, and when I came home in the evening Yolaine would serve me a fine meal of Provençal cuisine made with vegetables from our own garden, and then we would make love like peasants.

It was the week when, with all lingering ambivalence washed away and drowned in the soft Mediterranean surf, we resolved with hot certainty to marry. And it was the week when I first shared with Yolaine my private joy.

It was our second evening in Saint-Tropez and we were having dessert at a restaurant facing on the bay, when Yolaine said, "Richard, why are you always — I mean *always* — leaving the table? Every dinner, every night since I've known you, three or four times during a meal you leave, and then more times when we're at a disco. It is really very strange. Originally, you always said it was to go to the bathroom. And now it's to go to the bathroom *and* to make mysterious phone calls. In Washington and New York it was *dozens* of phone calls — and you don't even know anybody over here to call. *Nobody* has to go to the bathroom that much, no matter what their problem; and *nobody* has to make that many phone calls."

The time obviously had come. I smiled and said, "Well, what do you think it might be, my love?"

"I'll tell you *exactly* what I think it might be," she said in a tone that was at once triumphant and conspiratorial. "Carole and I talked about it after you left Teildras and we both came to the same conclusion. And after Washington and New York, and now here, I'm more certain than ever."

"Certain of *what?*" Was it possible that she had suspected all along? I doubted it; I was one of the lucky ones whose behavior didn't go bad on coke. But what if she had suspected? So what? My confirmation of her suspicions clearly wasn't going to be a trauma; her knowing smile was too soft, her eyes too bright.

"Well, Carole and I think you're involved in some very funny business — not amusing-funny, peculiar-funny. You keep talking about being a consultant, and I understand the part about lobbying the government. But there's a lot of what you describe that I really don't understand; it's both too vague and too complicated. When we were in the States, you ran off to little private meetings — very short meetings. And the endless private phone calls and bathroom trips — no matter what part of the world we're in. Carole and I think you're either involved with the Mafia or are a CIA agent."

Immediately she held up her hand, with her palm facing toward me, to forestall my response before it began. "No, wait, sweetheart. Before you say anything — anything at all — I want you to know that it doesn't matter, whichever it is. I'll marry you anyway. Although I would hope it's the CIA. Actually, I've always wanted to be a spy myself, and it would be awfully exciting to be married to one."

My first reaction was dumbfounded silence. Then I cracked up in waves of laughter that filled my eyes with tears. "Oh, Yolaine," I gasped, "you are wonderful, absolutely wonderful." And I thought to myself that it figured. The French — the wonderful French. They *lived* for intrigue; and if there wasn't any around, their fertile imaginations simply made it up. Yolaine had seen a lot of symptoms of apparent wealth since we had been together — mysterious wealth whose sources she didn't understand. And meetings, and obscure phone calls, and quick trips to latrines in the night. The French loved American movies, and the ones about rich Mafiosi and elegant spies were the ones they loved best.

"Oh, sweetheart, I wish it were only so," I said. "But I've got to disappoint you. Look, do you remember that first night in Paris, when I asked if you had ever tried cocaine?" — and I took both her hands in mine. "No, wait. Don't get upset. Wait until I've finished. I know how you feel about drugs. But you've got to understand that your brief experience in L.A. was with the wrong kinds of people. It isn't that way at all with a lot of good people — people who enjoy the effects of a little marijuana and cocaine, but keep their lives under control.

"Yes, that's what I'm telling you — the bathroom trips and telephone calls are to have a little cocaine. Do you remember all my friends at your house for dinner the night we met? Remember how much you liked everybody — their great sense of fun, and the energy of the night? Well, a lot of us were using coke. And were any of us monsters? Of course not, we all were just having a wonderful time. And, admit it, *you* thought we were wonderful.

"And all the time we've spent together — I've been using a little cocaine. Not much, understand, just a responsible amount. And how have I been — not bad at all, right? In fact, quite good. You've loved me. Respectable people in Europe have a very different idea about drugs than Americans — that's because you really don't know anything about them except what you see in movies. In the States, nearly all of my friends who have the money to pay for it use coke. Lawyers, bankers, media people — *everybody*. The *best* people use coke. I'm not talking about addicts. I'm talking about the *best* people — *responsible* people. Sweetheart, I would have told you sooner, but the time wasn't right."

It had been a long speech but a good one, and I felt relieved that it finally was on the table. Yolaine sat for a long time drawing circles with her fork on the table cloth. When she finally spoke it was without anger, but with a worried touch of sadness.

"Richard, you're right. I really don't know much about

drugs, but what I have seen has made me afraid of them. I don't judge you at all, but I'm afraid for you."

"Do you trust me?" I asked.

"You know I do. I'll trust you to the end of the world."

"Then try a little cocaine with me tonight. Just a little. You'll see."

And Yolaine did trust me, and she had some cocaine with me that night while we lay in bed, drinking a simple local wine. And for the first time we made love with both of us raised up to the sensual height that was cocaine's gift. And I was glad that at last we could share the experience that, for too long, I had had to keep secretly my own.

Each night thereafter we snorted cocaine together. I had a lot more than Yolaine, but she didn't need very much to get to feeling wonderful, and she had a rare capacity for self-restraint. She loved the drug and I loved sharing it with her. Driving away from Saint-Tropez, and up through Provence along the banks of the Rhône, we reminisced about our languorous days in the water and sun, and our nights of dining, dancing, and love. And we talked about the wonders of cocaine.

"Promise me one thing," she said.

"What's that?" I asked.

"That you won't use too much of that stuff. It is terrific, I admit it. But you should be careful. Promise me."

"I promise," I said.

Teildras was even lovelier that first week of September than it had been in June. La Comtesse's perennials were everywhere in bloom, business was brisk, and Le Comte's icy façade of three months past had thawed to reveal a man capable of warmth. My surmise had been accurate. He had been impressed with my return visit to Yolaine, and with her excited stories of my prosperous, well-positioned life in the States, and had started to think of me as not just Yolaine's consort but as, quite possibly, a family asset. No longer a nonperson, I now lounged comfortably in the salons of the great old house, reading a book and sipping tea, or strolled about the garden and the wooded park, at ease with the family and myself. If I hadn't completely arrived quite yet, I clearly was approaching the threshold of belonging.

On the second night of the five that I would spend at Teildras before flying back to San Francisco, Yolaine and I told her parents of our plans. She would stay at Teildras to help out until the season closed in November; then she would go to San Francisco to live with me. We would marry, but we weren't quite sure when; at the very least, we would wait out the year as I had promised.

La Comtesse raised her eyebrows, but gave Yolaine a smile and a mother's look of happiness for her daughter, however bizarre the circumstances. And Le Comte didn't protest at all, but merely shook his head knowingly and said, "Ah, oui," in the studied tone of a chairman of the board assenting to a sensible point well made by one of his directors. He had appraised the assets and liabilities of the liaison and, smelling American prosperity come to the family table, had managed to overlook the untoward appearance of his daughter living happily in sin for a while. Tacitly, we had come to understand each other.

Midmorning of the third day, I was sitting at a table underneath a big parasol on the terrace, drinking coffee and reading a two-day-old *Herald Tribune*, when Yolaine, who had been sleeping late, rushed up in her robe and gave me a kiss.

"Guess what?"she said excitedly.

"What, my love?"

"Fleur and Winfried are here! I had no idea they were coming. Mama said they got in after midnight. Fleur's still

218

in bed and Winfried's out fishing. Oh, isn't it wonderful? I've been dying for them to meet you."

Yolaine had gone on and on about Fleur, the middle sister who was two years older than she, and with whom she had shared many adventures and a special relationship. I had heard of Fleur's early wildness and incurable theatricality. Before she was twenty she had run off to Australia to live with a handsome commercial fisherman.

Another year, she had dyed her brown hair orange and had run off to Rome to become an actress. That career had gone nowhere, "But," Yolaine had said with an admiring laugh, "it did give her a chance to refine her natural sense of drama. With Fleur, everything — minor illnesses, little parties, shopping trips, passing flirtations — absolutely *everything* is a huge melodrama."

I had been warned that Fleur, at twenty-seven, was now in her "great lady" phase. Winfried, an international produce broker, had come down to Anjou from Cologne a couple of years earlier to make some deals on the coming apple crop, had met Fleur and married her. "Actually," Yolaine had said with a wink, "he would have asked any of the three of us. He liked the property. Anyway, he can be a lot of fun, and he and Fleur are perfect for each other. His money supports her marvelous pretentiousness, and he simply drools over Papa's title."

Winfried was a rich, self-made German who flew his own plane and had a taste for things French. And now Fleur was wrapped in furs, shopping exclusively at Yves St. Laurent, and, with her wild girlhood behind her, playing the refined-aristocrat role to the hilt.

I first saw Winfried at a distance, walking out of the thicket of woods at the far side of the meadow, where the river was. He had a fishing pole but no fish. When he got to the table he said, "I assume you are Richard," and said all the right things about how glad he was to meet me.

He was tall and lanky with a Prince Valiant haircut and a full beard that, on first look, gave him an impressive bearing, but that, on closer inspection, I thought had too obviously been shaped to give an illusion of strength to a weak chin. (It didn't occur to me then that if he had appraised my own beard, he might have jumped to the same conclusion.) He spoke English, I would learn, and four other languages fluently, but with a heavy accent. Even the most casual phrases were delivered in a tone of precisely clipped authority. And, in a classically German way, he kept repeating them as if, by the mere act of repetition, banalities could be transformed into great, authoritative ideas.

As we exchanged the obligatory pleasantries, it seemed obvious to me that, behind the heartiness, his nerves were wound tight and that he regarded me with as much suspicion as I regarded him. Whatever our eventual relationship was to be, at that first meeting we were prepared to see only the worst in each other. He went to great pains to emphasize "how happy Fleur and I are, Richard, to have you visiting in *our* house. It's too bad your stay has to be so short."

Fleur appeared on the terrace after lunch and she more than lived up to her advance billing. The only brunette among the daughters, she waltzed out into the sunlight perfectly coiffed and with taffeta billowing.

"I'm Fleur," she announced with a resounding ring of unabashed self-love that, in its airy enthusiasm, seemed not the least offensive.

"I guessed it," I said with a smile.

"Oh, Richard, you've made my little sister so happy, and she loves you, so I too love you. Well, don't just sit there; stand up and give me a kiss." I stood and she gave me a luscious kiss full on the mouth.

Putting a hand on each of my shoulders, she gazed intently into my face in mock-serious appraisal. "Richard,

Yolaine has told me *so* much about you." And then in a whisper, while wagging a finger under my nose, "Some of which a lady cannot possibly repeat in mixed company."

Her fluent English was spoken with a marvelous French accent that went well beyond the natural residual effects of her native tongue. It was an exaggeration calculated to charm the socks off Anglo-Saxons. Her every sentence seemed alive with hints of delightful innuendo.

"Winfried, why don't you go fishing again?" she said, gently waving the back of her hand at him. "I want to talk to Richard." And Winfried was only too glad to go.

"Winfried hardly ever catches anything except catfish," she said. "But it helps him relax. Now, tell me everything about yourself. What are your plans? When are you going to make my hot-blooded little sister a respectable woman?"

The afternoon passed in happy sunshine. Over cocktails before dinner, Fleur suddenly announced a big idea. "Richard, I have it! We're coming down here in October to baptize Friedrich at the village church. All of our friends are coming from Cologne, and we're giving a huge party afterward. A *fantastic* party. There will be people from Paris — and a few of the better ones from around here. Honestly, it is going to be *the* party of the year. You'll come. Yes, of course you will." I thought Winfried's face showed a deliberate lack of expression.

"Oh, Fleur, that's awfully nice of you, and I'd love to. But it's quite impossible. I've been traveling too much. I've got to do some work and—"

"Richard, that's a wonderful idea," Yolaine cut in. "Carole's birthday's in October and so is yours. The night after the party for Friedrich, we'll have another party for you and Carole. We'll have *two* parties."

"Fantastic," Fleur said. "*Absolutely* fantastic."

"Well, I don't know. I—"

"Oh please, darling. Think about it."

"All right, I'll think about it."

In bed that night, with pastries, champagne, and co-caine, I told Yolaine that Winfried seemed a basically nice fellow, but that our conversations had been strained. "On the surface everything was properly pleasant, but under-neath I felt some distinct unfriendliness."

"Richard, you've got to understand something. First, Winfried's German, and Germans are uptight to begin with. As a German, he feels both like a victim and a sinner. He's got a real identity problem.

"Until you showed up, Winfried was *the* man of the family in the next generation. There were no others. I know what he and Fleur have in mind, although they're too clever to talk about it. After Winfried makes his for-tune — frankly, I don't think he has the money he pre-tends to, but that's another question — they plan to live in Paris or New York and convert Teildras back into a great private house. They will be glamorous international jet-setters, and this estate will be their lovely country re-treat. My parents will be gently retired into a comfortable little apartment in the house, and Carole and I will have nice suites of our own for when we and our husbands come to visit; but Winfried and Fleur will *preside*.

"Well, that's *their* plan. And Winfried has invested a lot in making it happen. He's given Papa a lot of money to keep this place going, and has ingratiated himself into a good position with Papa. He figures that, with all the help he's given, Papa will have no choice but to leave the prop-erty to Fleur, or maybe even transfer it to her before he dies. And of course Fleur, with her flair for intrigue, is constantly trying to manipulate Mama to that end.

"As for Papa's intention, nobody knows. He's a clever old fox. He'll take money anywhere he can get it to keep Teildras going, let Winfried believe he's got the inside track, but not make a definite commitment on *anything*. He won't tell anybody his real intention. But I do know one thing. If it weren't for the money problem, there's no question that Papa would leave Teildras to me — with guarantees, of course, that my sisters would have free access here. He and I have a really special relationship, and he knows that I care more about the property emotionally than Carole or Fleur. And, of the three of us, he thinks I'm the least crazy. Which is not the same as thinking I'm completely sane," she added with a laugh.

"Anyway, now you come along. And you wonder why Winfried seems nervous and doesn't greet you with open arms? You look like you have money, and you're an *American*. And everybody knows that an American can pull off *anything*. Sweetheart, you're the new man on the scene, and Winfried sees you as a threat to everything he dreams about.

"But don't worry, you'll get to like each other. Winfried really has a generous, loving spirit, and you, of course, are hopelessly lovable. In time, I know that everything will work out as it should."

I swallowed hard. "How much money has Winfried put into the business?" I asked.

"I really don't know," Yolaine said. "But I think it's somewhere between fifty and a hundred thousand dollars, including the purchases he's made for the wine cave."

My throat had grown drier and drier with tension as I had listened to all of this, and I took down half a glass of champagne in a gulp. Over the past couple of months my own plans for Teildras had been taking a clear shape in my mind, and now it looked as though the whole wonderful scheme could be thrown out of whack by one overlooked but very large detail — Winfried. I hadn't planned to share my ideas with anyone, not even Yolaine, for a while, but now I felt a compulsion to accelerate the timetable.

"Sweetheart, let's have a little more coke. I've got something really important to talk to you about." And I dumped a big pile of powder onto the mirror on my lap and cut it into lines, and we each had a couple of big fat snorts of euphoria.

Confidence rushed up my nostrils, into my sinuses, and, in an instant, permeated my brain. Worry vanished as if by magic and my ideas took flight on words that soared into the room with a godlike precision and authority.

"Yolaine, I know how much you love this house and the land, and I love it with you. I know you want it, and I want it for you. But there is no way your parents can go on year after year with this operation — not the way it is. It's not just their age. The scale of the business is just too small ever to make money. They could have every room full throughout the season, and they'd never be able to do much more than pay taxes and overhead. Their fixed costs are simply too high compared to their revenues. Look at the staff — a maid, a gardener, a receptionist, assistant chefs, and two waiters, and all for a handful of rooms. Oh, you have to *have* that staff to maintain the incredible quality of the place. I know that.

"But you could serve three times Teildras's present capacity with only a small increase in staff. Expansion, that's the thing. The business has got to be dramatically expanded. But, better than that, there's a way to make an enormous amount of money from this property, keep it in the family, and make it an even more exciting place.

"You've got about two hundred acres of the most incredibly beautiful land I've ever seen. By American development standards, you could easily build two hundred condos, cluster them to preserve vast amounts of open space, and have a fabulous piece of work. But we wouldn't build that many — whatever number your father would be comfortable with. And they'd be designed on the outside much like the old Anjou farmhouses, only with a modern look, and inside they'd be luxurious."

I envisioned sandblasting the old farm compound and making it an elite seminar center, with a swimming pool in the courtyard in the middle. Down between the meadow and the compound, I'd put some tennis courts. We'd have one of the most attractive developments in Europe.

I figured that the condos would sell for between two hundred and four hundred thousand dollars. They'd be purchased by topflight people all over the world. Our family company would make a fifteen-percent commission on renting them out when the owners weren't using them. And that would be *on top* of the millions we'd make on the sale of the houses.

There would be seminars on the arts and on politics and on international politics, attended by the most important people in their fields in the world. As I described the plan, I could see Yolaine getting really excited.

"And the best part is that the house will become a family residence again. We'll still keep the dining room going — and it will be filled every night with the most interesting people alive — and the salons may be used for small seminars and cocktail hours. But the upper two floors will be divided into fabulous family apartments. The guests will stay in the condos.

"Teildras will become a center of intellect and culture, and the family will make millions in the process, Fleur and Winfried included. But we'll control the project. And your father will see the property become a living testament to centuries of de Bernard tradition. Well, what do you think?"

Her face was flushed and her eyes were dancing. She looked at me with something akin to awe. "I think it's absolutely the most fabulous thing I've ever heard," she said. "And Papa would love it; it would put him back where he thinks he belongs in life, and it would save the family."

"Not just *save* the family, Yolaine — make it *rich*."

"Could you really do all that, Richard? How would you finance it?"

"Simple," I said. "We'll form two organizations. The first will be a development company. I'll get the construction capital from investments in that company; I've got a lot of contacts in the investment community, and, with a really good plan, getting the money shouldn't be a problem. They'll put up the cash and your father will put up the land, and the investors and the family will split the profits from the condo sales fifty-fifty.

"Second, I'll organize a nonprofit foundation dedicated to educational purposes. That will be financed with contributions from major public-spirited corporations, whose executives will sit on the board of directors. We'll also put a university president and maybe a senator on the board. With that kind of letterhead, the foundation-sponsored seminars will attract the best people from everywhere — corporate executives, academics, statesmen.

"If I can get some kind of written agreement with your father that I can use to raise money in the States — not now, of course, but before long — I can *do* this thing, and it'll be terrific for everybody."

My weeks of nervousness about how and when to spring my ideas on Yolaine, without seeming too grasping, had been unnecessary. Cocaine was wonderful in its creation of instant understanding. She was with me every word of the way, her enthusiasm mounting with my every impassioned statement. I was not just her lover anymore, and her husband-to-be, but also a shining knight come as savior and guardian of her family. Hot-wired on coke and mellowed by champagne, we were certain it would be so, and we made love in a newer dimension of understanding and then fell into sleep wrapped in each other's arms.

When we awoke in the morning, the first thing Yolaine said, as though continuing an uninterrupted conversation, was "You know, Richard, if you really are going to accomplish this incredible thing, there are two things you've got to start working on very soon. You've got to figure out how you're going to handle Winfried. He's not going to take this scheme lying down, however much money he and Fleur might make out of it.

"And you've got to get Papa's absolute trust. I think he's getting to like you, but there's still a long way to go — particularly with what's at stake. With Papa sold on the idea — and on *you* — Winfried won't be a problem, however mad he gets."

"Well, what do you suggest?" I asked.

"Come back here for Friedrich's baptism in October."

"Now, look, Yolaine," I started out with some exasperation, "I keep telling you that I can't keep endlessly pouring money out for these trips. And you're going to be with me just a month later in November anyway. I simply —"

"Richard, it's important. I really think it is," she interrupted. "I wouldn't ask you if I didn't think so. Well, that's not true, I'd ask you to come back anyway. I can't wait until November to make love with you again." And she faked a pretty little demure look, then slipped into one of smart sophistication, and I didn't know whether the arched eyebrow signified that I had better return for the property or for the boudoir. It didn't matter which; I agreed.

Although I didn't know how I would finance still another trip to France — that would make three in five months on top of our fling in Washington and New York — the more I thought about it, the more sense it made. The Teildras development project, although it didn't exist except in my head and now Yolaine's, was no longer just an interesting idea. For me, it was rapidly becoming an absolute necessity. Despite fits of intense and productive work sandwiched in between my ocean-hopping, for the better part of three months I had been neglecting my clients, and I didn't know if I would even have any when I got back. It was a reality that I had kept pushed well back into the obscure recesses of my mind, but, even with the coke's ready reassurances, I couldn't ignore it any longer.

Still, the project was crucial. The *project* was *everything*. No longer was it just something that would be nice to do if I could manage it. Sometime in my sleep the truth had hit me, for I awoke in the morning to the startling realization that without the project — or without something very much like it — I was financially dead.

Everything had happened too fast, the whirlwind romance, the jet-setting. Through much juggling, I had been able to manage the financing — or at least to put off settlement to some seldom-thought-of judgment day in a hazy future. But suddenly I knew that that day had arrived. I was already technically insolvent and probably approaching bankruptcy.

The problem hadn't begun just with Yolaine. From the time of my separation from Arlene, when the parties had become more frequent, the cocaine more readily available, the mornings of sleeping in to recuperate more comfortable and less guilty, I had been cutting my work short. But I was good at what I did, and my income had continued to rise, although the increase had not matched the additional amounts spent on coke.

But the coke wasn't the problem either; I was sure of that. Indeed, the coke had been a real benefit. It had made me realize how mundane my professional life really was, despite its superficially glamorous trappings. I could get really creative on good cocaine. This wasn't the first great project it had helped me conceive; it was just the first one whose elements suddenly appeared in the palm of my hand. On good coke, my mind was a tornado of ideas, each better than the others, and with its help new visions of the possible had unfolded.

The only problem was the timing. I had, in mind and action, if not by way of formal announcement, simply abandoned professional boredom for a richer life a bit too precipitously. There was a "technical" problem with the financial transition, that was all. And I would solve it. I'd go back to San Francisco and raise some money for "the project," and work out the details with Le Comte later. Of *course* I would come back to Teildras in October for the baptism. It would be a prudent move business-wise. My love for Yolaine, "the project," my chivalrous instincts toward her family's salvation, and the urgent demands of my very survival, all merged into a wonderful, single, shining ball of wax, self-justifying and infinitely rational. I had some cocaine to get the day started.

The morning after my arrival back in San Francisco, I woke up flat broke. I didn't open any of my mail because most of it was from people like landlords, bank loan officers, utility companies, and other like-minded types looking for the money I owed them. There was also a letter from Philadelphia that I didn't open. The envelope bore my client's logo, and I knew the contents weren't glad tidings, but an outraged inquiry as to where I had been and what I had been doing for them in return for their money.

Instead, I made some coffee and went immediately to the typewriter to write a proposal amending my consulting contract with Mel's company. I read it over, pleased with the plausibility of my justifications for adding another twenty-five thousand dollars to my fees, and took a draft down to the local secretarial services to have it typed on my letterhead. That done, I drove into San Francisco to give the proposal to Mel.

He said he was glad to see me and looked over the proposal. "It looks fine to me," he muttered, and gave me a smile. He spread some healthy lines of cocaine out on his presidential desk, and we snorted and chatted warmly for a while.

"Come back around two o'clock," Mel said. "Go see

Phil, and he'll have a check for you. And I'll see you again in a day or two, won't I?" And another smile. I said that he would.

I picked up the check from the controller precisely at two, went to the bank and deposited it into my account, and withdrew two thousand against it. Then I drove out to Greg's and bought a quarter of an ounce for six hundred and twenty-five dollars, and paid off the eleven hundred I owed him. Two days later I drove out to Mel's house, had a little cocaine and wine with him, and gave him ten thousand in cash.

When I dropped by the bank again to see Frank, my loan officer, he had turned friendly again. "You don't know how relieved I was to see that deposit of yours show up on the printout," he said. "You know your overdraft had gotten up to about six thousand. I guess you're as glad as I am to see that wiped out. Now what about the loan?"

I gave Frank a few hundred dollars to take care of past-due interest, and told him that I still couldn't pay anything on the principal for a while. He didn't protest; he considered himself lucky. In forty-eight hours the twenty-five thousand that I had gotten from Mel had shrunk to under six thousand. But I was liquid again for a while, and I felt good about my situation. I had enough money to pay one of the two months' rent that was past due and, since my landlord lived in Los Angeles and didn't have a local manager, I could continue to string him along a month or two in arrears without getting kicked out. There was enough to pay the utilities and, if I was careful for the next month, I would still be in shape to finance the trip to Teildras for the baptismal party.

The hesitations of conscience about Mel's offer that, only a few weeks earlier, had caused me to postpone a decision had vanished. I had accepted the check from the controller without feeling a twinge of guilt. The only qualm I'd had when the big stack of new hundred-dollar bills had passed from my hand to Mel's in an envelope was over his unconscionable greed; the percentage that he was taking seemed grossly excessive by the usual standards that I assumed prevailed in such transactions. But I had been in a hurry to get my affairs in a semblance of order, and had been uninclined to argue with him. For my part, my services were worth a lot, and his company would get value for its money, however convoluted my means of getting paid. Besides, I reminded myself, we had clearly called Mel's money a "loan," hadn't we? If he chose not to repay, that was his ethical problem, not mine.

My behavior in such matters had gone through a subtle change, educated by the realities not only of business, but of life. I hadn't at all lost my idealism; if anything, my goals were more shining and worthier than ever. But, if you had talent and visions to fulfill, and didn't have money to begin with, there was hardly any way to bring life to fruition *quickly* without some compromises of middle-class conventions.

I consciously thought about ethical considerations less and less, but when I did, it was clear to me that *results* were what mattered, not the means for getting them. And everybody I was involved with *ultimately* would get *value;* that was the main thing, not the sleights of hand that might be required in the interim. Besides, I was sure that there was hardly a fledgling entrepreneur around who wasn't cutting corners more sharply than I was. If Mel and I had broken the law, it was, at worst, a *technical* breach of rules that didn't accommodate special circumstances and special people.

I had committed a felony each time I had bought some coke, each time I had carried it in my pocket, and each of the thousand times I had snorted it up my nose, over the past few years. Wasn't that proof enough of the stupidity of laws? The smartest, most successful people in the country were coke users. Did that make us a country of dangerous felons? Of course not. For years, anachronistic drug laws had forced me into a pattern of devious behavior and sneaking about and the habit of breaking *that* particular set of laws hadn't made me a bad person, but an infinitely happier and more creative one. Selective lawbreaking was no big deal if it served the justifiable needs of the *right* people. It wasn't a matter of criminality, but of *misunderstanding*.

If Mel and I were to use a substantial part of our spoils to buy more cocaine, that was no big outrage either. Cocaine helped refine dreams, and infused the brain with astounding ideas for achieving them. And, even when, because of technical impediments, the gratifications promised by the dreams had to be deferred, cocaine brought an instant gratification all its own. Instant gratification, that was the thing. And the holding out of endless promises for more. In the end, everyone in my world would be the better for it.

It was a relief to find out that I was still in my clients' reasonably good graces. They had been troubled about having been unable to reach me, but their concern had been much less intense than I had feared. I decided that I had started getting far too paranoid and resolved to check the tendency and get on with the adventures ahead.

I worked a bit during those weeks on my clients' affairs to keep them happy, and to build up a little bit of a financial cushion. But the truth was that I had lost all interest in the work. It was too detailed and too mundane compared to my grander ideas. So, having been unsuccessful in getting myself fired, I began gradually easing myself out of a professional career that had been twenty years in the building.

I spent a lot of time that September working on the Teildras development plan — conceptual design, cost and revenue projections, market absorption rates, tax consequences, sales strategies — all of the stuff that would go

232

into an elaborate package to impress Le Comte, and then the investors. That was the month when I started using cocaine not just for nighttime merriment, to get myself started in the morning, and for an occasional midday snort with a friend, but constantly when alone at my work. And it had some odd results.

When I was working on my regular consulting analyses and reports, the coke made them even more boring and inconsequential, and, when my nervous frustration exceeded toleration, I would put them aside. I'd return to them, I told myself, when I was in a better mood. But, when working on "the project," my brain soared. The calculator hummed, and the typewriter keys sang across page after page in a symphony of articulation, logic, and eloquent persuasion. The incredible promise *was there*, anybody could see it — in my own compelling words. I wrote and snorted, wrote and snorted. Never had I been so mesmerized by the clarity of my written thoughts, nor so certain of their infallibility.

I didn't finish the project proposal that September, but I got enough of it done to feel a new power. I had an escape into a paradise of my own making. And there was no need, really, to be overly fastidious about cultivating old securities until new ones matured. Old jobs were old jobs, and yesterdays were yesterdays — both to be put behind me as quickly as possible.

In October, the rains had come to France. In Anjou, the sky, the countryside, and the rivers were all colored the same leaden gray, and a cold drizzle saturated everything that moved. It was a different country.

But inside the château, the fireplaces were alive with burning logs and everybody was in a festive mood. That morning, Friedrich had been baptized in the decrepit old village church whose priests had blessed and buried generations of de Bernards. I was astonished to see how seriously the French take their baptisms; I had never seen such an elegant private party even for a rich adult on an important birthday, let alone for an infant. Fleur stage-managed it with theatrical flair, and Winfried paid for it, and I thought it a wonderful way for a family to celebrate itself on an occasion of new, and hopefully everlasting, life. It didn't occur to me until the next morning that there was something menacing to my interests about a male infant being brought by his German father all the way from Cologne to the tiny village of Cheffes in France to be baptized, about the child being given the de Bernard name, and about the lavishness of the party itself. The party wasn't just a celebration; it was a statement of presumptive proprietorship. The unknowing infant was being displayed by his father not just as another beautiful baby, but as the putative, if not openly proclaimed, future Comte de Bernard.

The celebrants were a mix of local gentry, aunts and uncles and cousins, sleek sophisticates down from Paris, and rich-looking business associates that Winfried had brought with him from Germany. During stand-up cocktails before dinner, Friedrich, cradled in his father's arms, was given his gifts. At the last minute in Paris, Yolaine had rushed out of the hotel to the city's elite infant shop to buy an expensive little suit, and when Fleur opened it and held it up for display, everybody said how adorable it was. But the Germans were the stars of the show, and their act had been saved for last. Otto, Winfried's closest friend, presented Friedrich with a Deutschbank bond whose value, at the exchange rate then, amounted to several thousand dollars. I was impressed and so was everybody else, particularly, it seemed to me, Le Comte.

Winfried and Fleur were exceedingly warm toward me, and said how grateful they were that I had come all this way to celebrate with them. I took it as a compliment that, at dinner, they seated me with Otto and his wife, Hildegard. If Nietzsche and Wagner had collaborated to select the perfect Teutonic supercouple, they would have chosen Otto and Hildegarde. Both were tall, with hair as gold as flax, and eyes of a clear, almost unsettling blue. They had the same prominent cheekbones, which made her beautiful and him ruggedly handsome. She was encrusted with diamonds, and he wore a dark silk suit. Both had just enough flesh on them to make them formidable but not fat. They were approaching fifty but were in wonderful shape.

Otto was said to be astonishingly rich. Throughout the evening he engaged me in much talk of international politics and finance. It was unclear exactly how he had made his money. Something to do with investments and tax shelter deals. And there had been some transactions in the Middle East, mentioned offhandedly and then dropped. Currently, he was involved in "something" in Central America. He said that Winfried had mentioned my political connections in the States, and that he was impressed. He said that, for a time, he had been a consultant to McNamara at the World Bank. Otto said that we undoubtedly would be seeing more of each other, and that maybe there would be a basis for him, Winfried, and me to do some business together. Hildegard said that they had a wonderful house in Port Grimaud, just across the bay from Saint-Tropez, and hoped that, if Yolaine and I got down that way again, we would feel free to use it.

It was a happy weekend. The next evening the family gave a joint birthday party for Carole and me, complete with one of La Comtesse's delectable cakes. The family — even Winfried — was extending me gracious acceptance, and I felt that Yolaine's parents' attitude of resignation was sliding into affection.

I was concerned about the obstacle that Winfried presented, all the more so since I was beginning to like him. The party, to my mind, had been a beautifully orchestrated power play. But he had taken pains to offer unspoken tokens of friendship, or at least clear hints of an invitation into alliance. And an alliance would be fine with me — far preferable to open warfare — but it would be on my terms. And I was confident I could make it happen. He might have more money than I — *how* much was uncertain — but *I* had the superior talent, and *I* had the proposal for "the project." And however much money he had available to put up for Teildras, I would have more — not mine, maybe; but plenty of other people's.

Yolaine and I talked about whether we should discuss my plan with her father, and decided that it would be prudent to wait until the proposal was completed and all the details were wrapped up in an irresistible package. Maybe we should even wait until we were married.

I was in a hurry to get something going, but the success of my last-minute transaction before leaving San Francisco had made me realize that I could generate the cash I needed to pursue "the project" even without having certain details taken care of. Only two days prior to my scheduled departure for France, I had been almost out of cash — despite a serious effort to be careful with my money. I had had to buy more cocaine than I had anticipated and, imprudently, had used cash instead of my credit with Greg.

It hadn't taken me more than a couple of hours to conceive and draft a two-page "Investment Agreement" for the sale of "interim" financing shares in the Teildras project. And my old friend Donald, a prominent lawyer for a number of public agencies, had been delighted to get my call inviting him to lunch at Scott's fish place, out on Lombard Street.

Donald had explained to me that, despite all the money he was making, he wasn't a speculator; he was careful with his money. But he had been moved by the story of my romance with Yolaine and our plans for marriage, and had been impressed by my plans for the property.

"Dick," he had said, "I've never done anything like this

with my money, but I'll take one of your seven-thousand-dollar shares. As far as I'm concerned, you're a miracle worker, and I would follow you anywhere." Donald and I had worked a lot together. He had always been amazed by my magical ability to generate millions of federal dollars where nobody else could, and his trust in me was infinite.

I had explained to him that, while I didn't quite yet have a deal with Le Comte on the property, I was confident that I would have it very soon. And, in any event, the agreement provided that the investor had an option, exercisable in six months, to get his money back with a twenty-percent profit, or let it ride. Unaware of my use of cocaine, Donald knew me as a man of talent and integrity. He gave me the money for Teildras "planning costs" with barely a second thought.

I was confident that more of the same kind of money would be available from other friends when I got back to San Francisco. The fact that I was already raising money for a project that the property owner didn't even know about yet wasn't all that important. And there really was no need to share that fact with Yolaine. I was confident of the ultimate result. "The project" would succeed, and my investors would be handsomely rewarded.

Yolaine was right; my coming back for the baptismal party had been a good strategy. Not the time for the big push; but an important time for just being around and becoming part of the family. I was intrigued by my meeting with Otto. If his references to his past were sometimes ambiguous, his easy show of wealth had been impressive. I had no idea what he had in mind for me, but was confident that he had another shoe to drop. The Teildras project, it seemed, might be just the beginning.

6
. . . and Promises to Keep

Yolaine and I were to be married in France on June 21, 1980, almost a year to the day after the waiting period I had promised Le Comte. Yolaine had come to San Francisco to live with me the previous November, and we had had a year of recharged romance. I had expected it to be a calmer time, when we would get to know each other in a more real way — responsibly, with the incredible whirl of fantasy put behind us. But her excitement at moving to her new second country had been as great as mine when I had found her in France; and we had started our new life together in the States in a spirit of absolute freshness, as though we were brand-new lovers.

My friends, who had met Yolaine when we were all at Teildras the previous June, had an insatiable urge to fete us. James and Catherine hosted a smashing welcoming party, complete with little American flags and French tricolors at each table, and we laughed in gay reminiscence of James's unsolicited brokerage of our first date in Teildras's kitchen. And Michael and Alice, and Mel and Nina, entertained us endlessly.

Two or three nights a week we would go over to the little French bistro, where we were in intimate rapport with a whole new bunch of friends. Yolaine and the proprietor adored each other. She told him when his food was bad, and they talked a great deal about Marrakesh, which Yolaine loved and where he claimed to have a mansion. She and Wilkes Bashford charmed each other nightly, and she was delighted with Willie Brown, the suave speaker of the California Assembly, and thought it amazing that a black could rise so high in American politics. She loved my eclectic group of friends.

I took her over to Greg's one night to buy some cocaine, and found the entire freak show in attendance — the two ex-wives and the live-in girlfriend, with all their eyes stoned vacant; Tommy the Thief fencing a stereo and shooting up in the bathroom; the owner of a mortgage company down on the peninsula who had started free-basing his cocaine and had gone temporarily broke, and was nervously trying to persuade Greg to give him some more on credit; the spacey carpenter; the once-pretty graphic designer, who had lost twenty pounds since I had last seen her and looked like a ghost; the three waitresses who had just gotten off their shifts and were pooling their tips to buy a gram. Everybody smoking pot, nodding their heads to the beat of the rock coming out of the speakers, and acting very cool while waiting for their coke deals to come down, while Greg was back in his "office" with the door shut, busily weighing out the stuff on his electronic digital scale, pouring the precise amounts into little, carefully folded paper bindles, and otherwise getting himself organized for a big business night.

When, some two hours later, we finally walked out into the brisk Sausalito air, Yolaine took a deep gulp of it, as if it were a life-saving medicine, and said, "My God, Richard, what was all that, and who are all those creepy people?

"Your friend Greg's all right. A little strange, but attractive and sort of amusing. But everybody else — my God, I just can't describe it."

I explained to her how, in Greg's business, he necessarily had a lot of contact with some hard-core drug addicts, but that had nothing to do with us. I assured her that I didn't spend much time there myself, just to get some coke once in a while, and, as for Greg himself, he was okay.

As it turned out, we spent more time there during those months than I would have liked. But we generally managed to schedule our visits to avoid the freak show. And Greg and Yolaine got to like each other, although she frequently cautioned that we shouldn't get in the habit of going over there too often.

One night, we dropped by about midnight to pick up some cocaine. Greg and his girlfriend were the only ones there. We had a hot tub with them, snorted piles of coke and smoked several joints, and Greg gave Yolaine her first hit of amyl. We drank a lot of wine and, with our heads spinning out, made love on Greg's floor and fell asleep there.

Driving home in the morning in the Porsche, Yolaine said, "You know, Richard, you're really amazing. You are totally at ease everywhere with every kind of people. You can bounce from a night in a Sausalito pad with a bunch of overaged hippies and spaced-out dopeheads, and then back again to a Nob Hill society party. You are totally adaptable to everything and everybody. You're a universal man, that's what you are."

I smiled and said, "Why, thank you, my love. Yes, that's what I am — a universal man. I guess I do like a lot of different kinds of people. And Greg and a *few* of his crowd are amusing in small doses. But that's not my world or yours; it's just a place to get some coke and have a little offbeat fun once in a while." And I made a mental note that I should cut down on the time spent with Greg and his Sausalito coterie. However amusing, they were losers. If my upscale friends could see me in that environment, it would blow their minds.

In early December, Fleur called Yolaine with the breath-taking news that she and Winfried would be in New York the following week, and would be thrilled if we could join them there for dinner.

We checked into the Regency since my account was still delinquent at the Sherry-Netherland, and I called Tom Brokaw to ask for his help in getting us reservations at La Grenouille. Even with decent advance notice, it was hard enough to get into New York's handful of truly elite restaurants on a Friday night unless you were a favored patron or a recognized notable. To be unknown, and to call the same day, would be simply to offer yourself up as the butt of a maître d's contemptuous joke. I explained to Tom the urgency of my putting on a show for my future brother-in-law, and he said his secretary would take care of everything.

She must have laid it on very thick. The maître d', whom I had never seen before in my life, greeted us effusively and said, "Ah, Monsieur Smart, what a *delight* to see you again. You really shouldn't stay away so long." And he seated us at the center table that every great restaurant reserves for its most luminous stars, where, throughout the evening, the captain, two waiters, and the maître d' himself hovered in attendance to Monsieur Smart's every desire.

Yolaine went home for Christmas. Back in San Francisco in the first week of the new year, she got a telephone call from Le Comte inquiring whether, by chance, Richard might be in a position to give him some temporary financial help. The payments on the mortgage that he had put on Teildras when they had converted it into a hotel were badly in arrears and he had some other pressing bills.

"What about Winfried?" I asked.

"Papa says Winfried's reluctant to put any more money in right now. Apparently he's in a tight position himself."

So, I thought, I had been right in my interpretation of Winfried's reaction when he had looked at the dinner check in New York — a barely disguised expression of shock followed by a fleeting, but distinctly angry, glance that accused me of having deliberately sandbagged him. I had suspected then that he didn't have nearly the money that he pretended, and now I was certain of it. It would be a great thing if, with Winfried's fortunes down, I were in a position to rush in to fill the breach at Teildras.

Yolaine didn't press the matter, but simply said that it would be nice if we could help Papa. We had some cocaine and wine and settled in for the evening to weigh the matter. About three A.M., the time at which we usually came to our best decisions, the answer became obvious. However difficult, we should give Papa some money. Not only was it the family thing to do, it would be a good strategy in the undeclared war of intrigue over Teildras. And, actually, I didn't think it would be all that difficult.

Donald, my first "investor," wasn't of a mind to put up any more money yet; he wanted to see how "the project" progressed. But his best friend was an independently wealthy coupon clipper with whom he played golf a couple of times a week, and Donald would see what he could do. Calvin and I liked each other immediately, we signed my "investment agreement," and he gave me fourteen thousand dollars.

"You know why I'm doing this, Dick," he said. "You seem like a great guy, but I don't know a thing about you. But I have complete confidence in Donald, and Donald has complete confidence in you — he says you're golden. And that's good enough for me."

I sent Le Comte ten instead of fifteen thousand, and specified it as a loan, instead of either a gift or an investment in the family company. I didn't expect ever to ask for the money back. But it would be a good tactic to put him on notice that, while I was generous and committed to the family, I was a tough-minded businessman and not a soft touch.

I used the rest of the investment funds to live on and to pay a few bills. With all my new entrepreneurial activities, my consulting income was down to under two thousand a month. I hadn't taken the trouble to form a company to receive the investments, or to open a business account separate from my own, or to set up an accounting system to separate personal and business funds. Those were petty details that I no longer had a taste for. Besides, there really seemed no need to be picky about where the funds were going; I was the promoter and manager of "the project," and entitled to use the funds for my own support while going about the project business. I knew that eventually I would sort out the finances, but there wasn't time now. On the rare occasions when I did start to worry about such matters, I would have a couple of snorts of cocaine and my thinking would become clear again.

Throughout the winter and spring, Yolaine and I planned and played, and played and planned. We talked endlessly about our wedding, where we would have it and whom we would invite, and what the menu for the lavish dinner would be. And we kept refining "the project," rethinking the convoluted strategies that would bring us all prosperity and happiness. We planned and schemed and reveled in our brilliance until the suns of countless mornings peeked above the hills across the bay. We repeated ourselves a lot, but cocaine tended to make that happen; and with each repetition the dreams glowed brighter, and the path showed itself more clearly. I was glad that Yolaine had come to trust me so completely in the matter of cocaine. It made our love even dearer, our talk wittier, and — as we focused nightly on the very serious and complicated business at hand — it made our heads ever-so-much clearer. Together, the three of us had an irresistible power, and we knew it.

* * *

In May, our euphoria was marred by my father's death.
Although he had been eighty-seven and had slowed down
a lot, he had retained his acute mind and dry, ever-ready
humor almost to the end. Only two months earlier I had
driven up to Modesto in the Central Valley, where he and
my stepmother were serving as missionaries for the Mor-
man Church, to tell him about Yolaine, and my plans to
remarry. It had been thirty years since I had started drifting away from the church that the Holy Spirit had told
him was the one true path to exaltation in the Kingdom
of God, and fifteen years since I had told him that my
break with the family's heritage of faith was definitive,
and my apostasy had caused him much pain.

But, strangely, with the sharp cut of the umbilical cord
had come a relief from years of ambiguity, and in that
relief Dad and I had become spiritually closer than we had
ever been when I was young and, presumably, had shared
with him a common God. We hadn't seen each other much,
no more than once or twice a year. But when we had, he
had always taken great pride in my achievements. He had
been thrilled when I told him about Yolaine, and had joked
that he had always known that I would be the one to marry
the family into the aristocracy that was our proper place.

When I had seen him in Modesto he had been in good
spirits, but he told me he had been having dizzy spells.
The doctors had detected a small cloudy spot on the front
of his brain.

Three days before he died, my eldest sister, Margaret,
had telephoned me from Reno, where he and my stepmother had their regular residence, and told me that I
should come because Dad had been asking for me.

When I got to the hospital he was in a coma, but recognized my name and said it himself several times. Margaret told me that the previous night, when he had first

become comatose, he had for hours talked pleadingly to his mother, as though he saw her in Heaven, telling her that he had tried to do his best, had tried to live a good life, and asking her forgiveness, love, and help. I was surprised and saddened that my father, whose life had been a dedicated example of rectitude and piety to his children, should, as he died, have had to suffer the remorse that afflicts ordinary men, and an agony of uncertainty as to his worthiness to enter the Kingdom of God. Then I remembered the times when, in his futile efforts to buttress my faith, he had confided his own doubts, his own lapses of faith, his own lifelong fears that he wasn't "measuring up."

Of all the men I had known, Dad had seemed the most deserving of that serenity in dying which is the reward of saints. And I was puzzled and sad that his death had been so hard.

My brothers and sisters asked me to give the eulogy at the funeral, and I was deeply touched. Their request that I, the only prodigal among them, be the one to honor our father's life, was a gesture of love that filled a felt hunger. Despite the many years that I had been separated from the faith of my brothers and sisters — a faith in which church meant family, and family meant church — they had retained a deep affection for me, and I for them. And I wanted to end my habitual inattention to my brothers' and sisters' lives; I wanted to reconnect with them in a meaningful way, and become again, as I had been as a boy, a part of a *family*.

"Family" was an idea that, over the years, had become for me an affectionate afterthought, to be indulged on the rare occasions of reunions and at Christmas card-writing time, but not a thought that I permitted to intrude upon the real — the *important* — priorities of my high-powered life. But, with my discovery of a new love with Yolaine, and with my witnessing of the closeness of her family, I had experienced a rekindled desire for my own. My father's funeral, and my family's request that I speak, would be, for me, a profound new beginning.

Mormon funerals are virtually unvarying in their themes — much bearing of witness that the church is the exclusive path to godliness, praising of the deceased's righteousness in faith, and invocations of the sacred obligation to likewise honor God. But my eulogy would be different; I would tell the truth as I saw it, without either sentimentalizing my father's life, or paying hypocritical homage to a view of God that I didn't share.

I spoke not of my father's apparently easy saintliness, but of his doubts and conflicts, and his lifelong fight to overcome them; not of his piety and rectitude, but of his love and understanding for a prodigal son who could not share his beliefs. I said that my father's life was not a testimony to the easy grace of God, but to the dignity of his struggle with himself. I said that, if he died a saint, it was not because he had always had a certitude of faith, but because of the nobility of his battle to overcome doubt.

And my brothers and sisters, and the hundreds of mourners who had known my father, were moved to honest tears, and I was lauded for a beautiful eulogy.

I was acutely sensitive that day — to the occasion, the environment, and memories of the past. I felt a love for my brothers and sisters that transcended all that separated us. They had all become prosperous through years piled upon years of methodical, hard work. Tom was a physician and Bill a newspaper editor, and Margaret had married a business executive, and Mildred, a dentist, and twice-widowed Mary, a nuclear physicist and then an entomologist. They had devoted their lives to stability and what the upper-middle class defines as responsibility, and I had devoted mine to risk-taking adventures. I was sure that none of my brothers and sisters had ever cheated on their spouses, for they were all devout Mormons, and the

246

church proclaimed adultery a sin second in gravity only to murder. They knew nothing of the voluptuous delights of sex on Quaaludes, or the fun rush of a snort of amyl in a hot tub, or the heady bouquet of a fine Bordeaux at Maxim's. They got their satisfactions in more prosaic ways — working their way up to solid houses in which they raised large families of disciplined children whom they sent to college; taking one or two modest vacations a year in quiet, family-type places; saving money for their old age and for their children; paying their bills on time. And worshiping — *always* worshiping — God.

The church building brought back memories of so many other, almost identical, churches in which I had spent my childhood. They all evoked, in their forthright simplicity, the character of the people who built them. Brick, always brick, with a semblance of a steeple but no cross. Churches like this were a far cry from the great cathedrals of Europe that I had come to love so much, or from the church in Anjou where Yolaine and I would be married in only a month. There were no candles, no priests and altar boys in ornate robes, no trappings of religious theater. The starkness of the building, the solid, open faces of the people and the plain clothes they wore were at once a pageant of my past and a reminder of how far I had come.

On the flight back to San Francisco, after a Bloody Mary and some cocaine, I thought how wonderful it would be if I could share some of my new life's good fortune with my own family. When the time was right, I would give them an opportunity to invest in "the project." They were all successful in their own right, but this would be different. They would share in the fruits of *my* success — the prodigal's success — and that would bring us an even greater closeness and love in a new direction.

The week before I was to leave for France — Yolaine had gone on before me to prepare for the wedding — I was faced with a crisis. I had expected Calvin to let his project investment ride for the duration; but he told me that he had to exercise his option to pull his cash out, so he could use it for an apartment house he was buying. With the profit I had promised, I had to come up with twenty thousand dollars. On top of that, I had had some unanticipated costs, and I was broke. I was supposed to be getting married in two weeks, and I didn't even have money to get there. In a panic, I called Michael and told him that I needed to borrow thirty thousand dollars for sixty days. He wasn't enthusiastic.

I cajoled and begged and persuaded, and finally said, "Listen, Michael, if you don't loan me this money there isn't going to *be* a wedding," and he relented.

"But I'm not going to loan you the money directly," he said. "I've got too many of my own cash needs. But I'll guarantee a note for you. And look, Richard, you and I both know you aren't going to have the money in sixty days, so let's make it six months. Don't leave me hanging out on this." Michael was worth millions and I knew that his guarantee was as good as gold. I met him at the bank and had the money in two hours. I was still living from crisis to crisis, but I knew that that was just a symptom of aggressive entrepreneurship. I bought more cocaine from Greg that night, and felt possessed of a power to achieve all things.

Yolaine and I were married in a tiny fifteenth-century church in Behuard that had literally been carved out of a stone cliff, adjacent to a monastery. Well, "married" is not quite the word for it. We had had the civil ceremony required by French law in the morning at the office of Cheffe's mayor. Even though the kindly old village priest had tried his best to get a special dispensation to marry us in church, the request had been denied on two grounds — my divorce and my Mormon baptism. But, in the interviews, the priest had seen how much we loved each other, and touched by the spirituality of our union, had promised he would do something special and very holy.

He gave a beautiful speech about the sacredness of marriage and the holiness of love, based on our answers to questions that he had put to us. And through it all, Yolaine and I sat in chairs before the altar, on a platform raised above the congregation, she in white lace, and I in a gray morning coat, while a choir of young people celebrated our love in joyous Latin hymns. Their songs rose to the ancient vaulted ceiling and echoed down upon us, while the flames of candles flickered in tempo to the music. When the Eucharist was offered, every Catholic went to the altar, even those who hadn't been in church in years. Afterward, many sophisticates who prided themselves on the anti-clericalism that pervades the French educated class, told us how moved they had been by the holiness of the occasion.

I felt immersed in history and God, and knew I was where I belonged. I stole a look at Michael — the ultimate sophisticate — and saw him with moist eyes, holding Yolaine's mother's hand. I had never felt closer to my best friend. In the last nervous hours of my bachelorhood, we had spent the morning together in my room, getting dressed, drinking cognac, and snorting cocaine. And although neither of us qualified for the Eucharist, our own sacrament had raised us together in a communion of the spirit that no holy wine could offer.

The church ceremony had been confined to family and very close friends. But the evening at Teildras was an immense celebration. Local aristocracy and business friends, gallery owners and bankers from Paris and an editor of *Le Monde*, the mayor, and Yolaine's childhood friends and sweethearts, including the boy from across the meadow — now a Paris banker — with whom La Comtesse had once caught her playing doctor. There were Belgians and Englishmen and Germans and Americans; and wine and champagne and music and buffet tables heavy with food. There were hundreds of lively, happy, substantial, celebrating people. And, again, I knew I was where I belonged.

Yolaine had never been more beautiful, running about in haughty grandeur, proud of herself and her man. Once she pulled me aside from the happy bedlam and whispered, "Oh, Richard, do you know how much I love you? It has been years since my parents have seen anything like this. For so many years they've worked so hard just to stay afloat. Now Teildras is a happy place again — because of us!"

About nine o'clock the family began a delicate exercise — getting rid of the people who had been invited just to the reception, and whispering discreetly to the chosen that they should stay on for more festivities. And, with the chaff separated from the wheat, the second chapter of celebration began — a sitdown dinner for the hundred who remained, served by tuxedoed waiters, with the best of champagnes and the most delicate of cuisine. And the jazz band played until five in the morning, and we danced all night. Donald, although he could speak only a few words of French to the band members, sat in at piano. I hadn't been able to return his "interim" investment in "the project," but he wasn't worried at all. With the joy of friendship, he had accepted my invitation to come and play at my wedding.

Late at night, Le Comte took me aside and told me how proud he was to have me in the family, and I remembered that I had never asked him for his daughter's hand. I did so then, after the fact, and he let forth a roar of a laugh that I had never heard from him before, and haven't heard since.

We honeymooned in Saint-Tropez, in Otto and Hildegard's luxurious house at Port Grimaud. Hildegard had been delighted when Yolaine had telephoned to inquire whether her offer to me at Friedrich's christening dinner was still good, and had insisted that we use their boat as well. Otto was out of the country, but she said he would be delighted to know that he had been able to contribute to our happiness.

Every day we had breakfast on the terrace and listened to the water lapping against the dock while we loafed in the gentle warmth of the morning sun. When noontime approached, we would hop into Otto's high-powered open boat and roar out into the bay and then into the Mediterranean, where we would anchor the boat and wade in to the beach to lie in the sun, kiss in the surf, and drink champagne at the outdoor café. Every night we danced, and one night we drove to the hills above Cannes to dine at Mougins.

We arrived late, but the proprietor kept the kitchen open for us because he knew Yolaine's parents, and, by special dispensation, we dined alone together in what many believe is the finest restaurant of France.

It was a time of tenderness and adventure. Careless of energy and time, we were fueled by the excitement of our love, and by the magic of cocaine. I had been close to running out, but, as one good friend was saying goodbye, he slipped a quarter of an ounce into my hand. It had been the most thoughtful of gifts. However burning our love, it would make our honeymoon infinitely better.

The night before we were to leave Saint-Tropez, a phone call came that we had been warned about. When Hildegard had told Yolaine that we could use her house, she had closed the conversation by saying, "Oh, by the way, if anyone calls, or drops by, looking for Otto, just tell them that you don't know where he is." Her offhand tone had seemed a bit too studied, but the instruction had seemed easy to follow since I barely knew Otto, and his affairs weren't my business.

Winfried had also taken me aside to emphasize the importance of Hildegard's instruction, and had told me that Otto was in Costa Rica. "His business there is confidential and very important — in fact, it's my business too — and nobody should know he's there. Otto's got some problems with the German government. Nothing that he won't get worked out, you understand — a misunderstanding, really. But for now, nobody — absolutely *nobody* — is to be told where he is."

I had put the warnings out of my mind until I picked up the phone and heard the voice say, "Doctor Otto Stern, *bitte*," and then a light clicked on in my brain and I was hit with a sudden case of nerves. I had been expecting a call from my two daughters who, after the wedding, had taken off with Michael's children on a tour of France; and, in my rush to shift mental gears, I faltered with a halting and, I knew, unconvincing response.

"Uh, who did you say, please?"

The German voice shifted to a precise but heavily accented English. "Doctor Otto Stern. I must speak to Doctor Stern immediately."

I explained to the voice that Otto was not there, that we were using the house with his wife's permission, and that I had no idea where he was. The voice didn't believe me. He repeated the urgency of contacting Otto and warned that "very large interests are at stake."

I again claimed ignorance in the most authoritative voice I could muster, and suggested that he try to reach Mrs. Stern at their Paris apartment. He said he had already talked to her and had gotten no information. The voice muttered something in German that sounded threatening and hung up.

I told Yolaine about the upsetting call. She said that it was nothing to worry about. "Otto's involved in a lot of huge deals, and it probably was just one of his business associates trying to reach him."

"Then why all the secrecy?"

"Oh, I don't know. He's probably doing something confidential, and just doesn't want anybody to know until he's got a deal concluded."

I was doubtful of that. "That voice sounded very official," I told her. "I'd bet anything he was from the Ministry of Justice or some other government agency."

"Well, what if he was? None of that has anything to do with us," she said; and I supposed she was right.

We decided to spend that last evening in Otto's luxurious house. I bought a bottle of fine Bordeaux, and Yolaine cooked a steak au poivre. Otto had an elaborate television setup that we hadn't paid any attention to, since we had spent all of our nights out on the town. He had a cabinet full of video cassettes and, in examining the inventory, I found a huge cache of porno tapes.

"My God, Yolaine, come and look at this," I said. "There must be over a hundred."

We looked at each other for a moment, then Yolaine giggled and said, "Let's." She had never seen a porno film and could hardly wait.

We had a lot of cocaine and wine and watched a provocative piece of highly artistic trash. And soon we were making love on Otto's deep-pile carpet, as erotic moans came out of the speakers, all the more arousing for their German accents. Whatever he was up to, and whatever his troubles, Otto Stern was a fascinating man of many parts.

When we got back to Teildras, Winfried and Fleur were still there. Winfried said he wanted to talk to me about a business proposition that he thought might interest me. We went into the salon at the far end of the house, where the walls full of books were.

"Richard," he said, "there are some exciting things going on, and Otto and I think you should be included. You're part of the family now, so I want to share some business opportunities with you, and I hope you would feel the same toward me. Do you know what I mean?" I allowed as how I knew what he meant.

"Otto is very impressed with your background. Last October when he had dinner with you, he liked you very much. He thinks that in what we're about to accomplish, it would be good to have an American contact, and I agree with him. Richard, we would like you to be the man."

I told him that I was very flattered, but didn't know anything about what they were trying to accomplish, or what they wanted "their man" to do.

"As you know, I've had a lot of experience in the international produce business, and I've spent a great deal of time in Latin America," he informed me. "And Otto's done some incredible things in finance. We've decided to go into business in a big way in Costa Rica.

"There are a lot of pieces in our plan, but the first thing — the fulcrum of our operation — will be a soybean processing plant. There's a great demand in Central America for high-protein animal feed and for vegetable oil for human consumption, and soybeans are one of the best sources of both. At present, the soybean meal and the oil are imported in finished form from the United States, and that's very costly. What we're going to do is import the raw beans and manufacture the meal and oil down there. We'll not only sell it in Costa Rica, but export it throughout all of Central America. It'll be a great thing for Costa Rica's economy, and we'll make a fortune."

"So what has Otto got to do with all of this?" I asked.

"Otto's there now, handling everything on the scene — you know, local planning, and arrangements with the government. He's got a tremendous amount of money and a lot of influence. Right now, he's working on getting us an exclusive license from the government that will give us a monopoly."

"So why are his whereabouts such a big secret?" I asked.

"Well, part of it is just a need for business secrecy, so somebody else doesn't try to cut the deal out from under us. But look, let me be frank. As I told you, Otto's got some problems with the German government. Some tax misunderstandings. But the government's wrong, and Otto's going to get the problem cleared up."

"And, in the meantime, he's found Costa Rica a congenial place — like Vesco?" I asked.

At my mention of the American fugitive whom the United States for years had been trying to extradite, first from the Bahamas and now from Costa Rica, for stealing two hundred million dollars in a securities fraud, Winfried's jaw tightened.

"No, *not* like Vesco. Otto's not a crook; he's simply got a problem." For all his pains to play the sophisticate, Winfried had little capacity for guile, and it was clear he believed this. "And in the meantime, he's made some very powerful friends in the Costa Rican government."

Whatever the truth about Otto, Winfried plainly trusted him, and was convinced they were embarked on a legitimate venture that would make an awful lot of money. I could make a judgment about that later, and for the moment take Winfried's statement at face value. If it turned out that he was naïve about Otto, that would be understandable; I had met Otto only once and had been thoroughly captivated by the man's charisma.

"Look, Richard, the soybean plant is only the beginning. We've got a huge real estate development on the drawing board, and we're going to buy coffee plantations. There are only about two million people in the whole goddamn country, and we're going to be the biggest force there."

"What do you want me for?" I asked.

"Eventually, we'll be doing a lot of business with the States, and you've got some valuable political contacts that could be useful. My lawyer in Cologne and I are putting the finishing touches on an investment package that we'll use in Europe. The great majority of the money will be raised here, but we'd like to get some American capital involved too. We'll pay ten percent on everything you raise."

"How much do you need?" I asked.

"We're raising, in dollar terms, about twelve million for the soybean operation, and we'd like to see two to three million of that come from the States. But here's the thing. Otto's got a big meeting scheduled in Costa Rica in a few weeks. I want you to come down there and see what we're doing. Important government people will be there, and the vice-president of a big multinational agribusiness who's involved with us — on a confidential basis, of course. It's really going to be fantastic."

I told Winfried that I'd be happy to go if somebody would pay my expenses but that otherwise I couldn't afford the trip. "Oh hell, Richard," he said, "we are talking about making some real big money. Pay your own way down there and get together with Otto, and we'll work something out. The important thing is that you get involved with us now."

Yolaine wasn't enthusiastic about the idea, but I persuaded her that it would be in our best interests for me to go to Costa Rica and get in on the ground floor of whatever was going on. She couldn't join me in the States anyway for about a month, since, in my preoccupation with the planning of the Teildras project, I had neglected to file some papers necessary for her admission into the States as a resident alien. During that time, I'd meet up with Otto and Winfried, and raise some money to support my participation in the venture when I got back to San Francisco.

I didn't entirely trust Winfried's judgment, but he seemed to know what he was doing, and he had been very persuasive. And Otto was a man of talent and intellect, not to mention great wealth. It was not just his manner and clothes and elegant Saint-Tropez house that were impressive; the photograph on the wall, of his sixty-foot power yacht, had spoken more eloquently of the world he commanded than anything Winfried had to tell me. I looked forward to the time when I, too, would be photographed on the deck in a blue blazer, alongside Otto, holding a very cold martini. Or maybe on my own comparable boat. My life was moving fast. The Teildras project would make Yolaine and me rich; and, if the Costa Rica potential was anything like Winfried had represented it, we would be rich beyond our wildest dreams.

I went back to San Francisco for a few days before going to Costa Rica. I had to buy some tropical clothes and some cocaine, and telephone the man whom Winfried had told me to contact to make arrangements.

I was to refer to Otto as Pedro, for he had obtained Costa Rican citizenship and was known there as Pedro Gonzales. His local partner, a man said to have irresistible influence with the government, was one Manuel Gonzales. Manuel and his wife had adopted Otto as their son, which is how he had obtained instantaneous citizenship. At least that was the story. And if people thought it quaint that a fifty-year-old man should put himself up for adoption, particularly to parents roughly his own age, nobody thought it shocking, for, as I would observe at first hand, Otto, a.k.a. Pedro, had the run of the country, and was a man much admired in high places.

When I got Manuel on the telephone, he was effusive in his greeting, and said that he was looking forward to meeting me, since Pedro had told him so much about me, and he knew how important I was to their plans. He asked what I would be wearing and said he would meet me at the airport.

The air in San José was hot and muggy. The flight from San Francisco to Miami and then on to Costa Rica had been long and tiring, and standing in the customs line I was sweating heavily and feeling very anxious. The customs people were passing some people through with no more than a perfunctory glance at their opened luggage, but others were being subjected to exhaustive searches that included every sock and piece of underwear; and I couldn't figure out what it was about some travelers that made them exempt, while others were viewed as presumptive smugglers. I was worried because I had a bag with a few grams of cocaine wrapped in a sock.

I was just stepping up to the customs desk, when a voice called out, "Mr. Smart — are you Mr. Smart?" I said that I was, and my greeter said, "Aha, I thought so; the description of the beard and sportcoat were very good." He flipped open his wallet and showed the customs agent a credential, then came through the gate, grabbed one of my bags, and said, "Come on, we don't fool around with any of this bureaucratic nonsense."

Manuel Gonzales was excessively unattractive. He stood maybe five-foot-six and had oily, reddish-brown, plastered-down hair that might have been a toupee in need of a wash, and the shoulders of his baggy polyester suit were covered with dandruff. In his lapel was stuck a large flamboyant pin, shaped like a royal crest and studded with diamonds. His face was ashen white, with a thin layer of sweat, and he had beady eyes that never settled in one place.

All the way into town, he rambled on endlessly about his wonderful country — its high literacy rate, its low crime rate, its work ethic, how much the poor loved the government, and how, while there were too many poor, none of them were dirty. None of it would have been offensive except that all of it came out in an obsequious whine. That, and his constant repetition of how wonderful the "projects" were going to be for the country, and, "of course" — with a mincing smile and insufferable oiliness — "for us." *This*, I thought to myself, is Otto's invaluable Costa Rican partner? I couldn't, for the life of me, figure out why a man of Otto's intellect and style would take up with this kind of company.

I soon found out why. Manuel's house on the outskirts of San José was a monument to ostentatious excess; wealth and bad taste were everywhere. Otto apparently had decided to overlook the bad taste and go for the wealth, or at least the influence and contacts that had created it.

I was ushered in through the entry by the pool and found myself in a huge sunken living room with twenty-foot-high walls and a balcony at one end. Above us there was no ceiling at all — only a blue sky with puffs of clouds. Winfried, Otto, a multinational agribusiness vice-president, and Winfried's German lawyer were huddled over a stack of papers at a long ebony table; and Winfried and Otto jumped up and gave me big hugs and introduced me to the others. Otto apologized that they had a couple of hours of intensive work to do, and Manuel said that he would amuse me in the meantime.

Another man walked in from outside, whom I was surprised to see. Alex was a Mexican — the son of a rich American father and rich Mexican mother — whom Winfried had introduced to Yolaine and me in New York as a dear friend and sometime business associate. He apparently was in San José as part of Winfried's deal, and I was reminded of the wag who had observed that there were really only sixty people in the world. I felt very much like one of them.

Alex and I exchanged warm hellos, and Manuel said we would have some drinks while the others worked and he would show us his collection of watches. Alex and I rolled our eyes at each other in an unspoken agreement that the man was a bore.

Manuel's houseboy brought in our gin and tonics in crystal stemware that sat on a silver tray. While we were drinking, I felt water falling on my head. Manuel looked up and said, "The afternoon rains, no problem," and walked over to a console where he pushed a button; there was a low humming sound, and, like a great white cloud, a ceiling came out of the top of a wall and moved slowly across the room until the sky and rain were gone.

"Let's go into the other room anyway," Manuel said. "I think you'll find it interesting, and I can show you my watches there." He picked up a polished mahogany box and led us into the adjacent room. It was like being transported through a time machine into the court of Louis XIV. The room we had been in before had looked like something a drunken interior designer with an unlimited budget had cooked up from a warped vision of the twenty-first century. Where we were now looked like an antique auction at Christie's.

Priceless antiques were everywhere. I was no expert, but the richness of the hand-turned wood proclaimed their authenticity. And everything — the tables and chairs and love seats and armoires and credenzas and breakfronts — *everything* was inlaid or leafed with gold. Not gold paint; gold *leaf*. There were gold and crystal figurines and gold loving cups and gold ashtrays and gold cigarette boxes. That room alone had to be worth millions.

I walked around the room carefully examining pieces while Manuel beamed. It was plain that, while they were genuine, on many of them the ornate, molded gold contours had been added, centuries after their manufacture, for effect.

Manuel sat down at one of his French tables and unlocked the mahogany box. Inside were about a dozen large, very old, gold pocket watches, all with beautifully etched covers over their faces, that popped up when you pressed a latch button.

"They're magnificent," I said. "Do they work?"

"Do they *work*?" he exclaimed. "Oh, yes, they work,

all right. Watch this." And his voice was dirty and con-spiratorial.

One by one, he took each watch and wound it and pressed some hidden part. And one by one, each started ticking, and, in most, little bells started ringing, and from each one of them, to the rhythms of the ticking and the bells, incredibly tiny gold figures emerged and moved vig-orously in various postures of fornication, fellatio, and cunnilingus.

I had not known that, in other times, the idle rich had commissioned great artisans to manufacture pornographic pocket watches. "How much are they worth?" I asked. The man was so gross that I cared nothing for subtlety; and I knew that he would be thrilled by the question.

"I can let you have the least of them for ten thousand dollars," he minced.

"No thanks," I said. "I was just curious."

As we left the room, I stopped at the doorway and looked back in. It was an odd place. Taken separately, each piece was a thing of extraordinary beauty. All to-gether, the scene was grotesque. If there was such a thing as too much, the remedy was not modesty of acquisition, but good taste. Manuel, for all his oiliness, was a man to be reckoned with; but I would do my own house differ-ently.

Manuel hosted a big party that night, and the offensive room became the stage for elegance. Everybody in the San José establishment was there — cabinet ministers, the vice-president, the son of the president, American and German businessmen, sophisticated young lawyers. And the women. All of the women were beautiful. They wore delicate lace and genuine jewels, and — to my astonishment — half of the beautiful women and handsome men were speaking *French*.

That night, Costa Rica was explained to me. There were practically no Indians there — less than three percent. It

261

wasn't clear, somebody joked, whether the Mayans hadn't gotten that far south, or whether they had all been killed off by the Conquistadors; in any case, they weren't a factor. Amidst all of the turmoil that was going on in the rest of Central America, Costa Rica was a bastion of sanity. A place where *anybody* could do business. And the country was a great friend of America, and the son of the president was delighted that I was there, because we could do business. It was sort of like Switzerland, somebody said. A place to do business, whatever side you were on.

All of the fifty or so people in the room were elegant and charming, Manuel excepted, and I could have been at a party in Paris or Rome. Off in a corner, I asked Winfried about Manuel, who spoke English with an unplaceable accent. I learned that Manuel originally was an Alsatian, but Winfried didn't know when he had come to the country.

I asked how he managed to get all these political and social heavyweights to come to his party, and Winfried explained that, through his contributions of political funds, Manuel was a major force in the country, and probably the single most important person in "arranging things."

"Well, how does he make all his money?" I asked.

"Basically, he buys and sells jewelry and gems."

At that, my eyebrows raised in skepticism. "Oh, come now, Winfried, you don't believe that he's bought all this with the income of a San José jeweler any more than I do. Tell me something. We already know that he arranged a convenient home for Otto in his troubles, don't we? Did he also arrange Vesco's sanctuary?"

"Oh, he probably knows Vesco, but I wouldn't know anything about that," he said brusquely. "I've got to go visit with the guests," and he abruptly walked off.

Manuel may or may not have brokered the Vesco deal with the government, and he may have had a nice little jewelry business, but of one thing I was certain: He was first and foremost a fixer, and he had done very well at it indeed.

All of the important guests went out of their way to seek me out. "Pedro" had explained to everyone that I had important contacts in the U.S. government, and access to investment capital, and the San José establishment was most solicitous.

It was evident that Alex and I had been brought to the country for a purpose beyond our orientation regarding the projects. We were part of "Pedro's" carefully staged dog-and-pony show for the local political gentry. The more people he could bring in from around the world, the greater the appearance of the project's reality. An American with political influence and access to money was an impressive part of the cast.

Otto's promotional theater was perfectly okay with me. In entrepreneurship, promotion is *everything;* if it's good enough, the theater becomes reality. And I could play that game as well as anybody.

For three days we were players in a hectic pageant of meetings with government officials, planning sessions, tours of property, elaborate dinners, and late-night drinks. I was glad I had plenty of cocaine, for it gave me more energy than anybody else, and a razor-sharp mind. Otto was particularly impressed with my quick grasp of large concepts, refinements of his ideas, and powerful articulation.

We worked on the financial package for investors in the soybean oil plant, and I suggested some important changes in the draft contract with the equipment manufacturer. Otto took us to meet with his local architect, who showed us a site plan and architectural designs for the real estate development. Otto explained that, for those rich foreign home-buyers who wanted them, Manuel could procure Costa Rican passports, which would be an appealing part of the package for many people. I didn't completely understand why a normal person would need two passports,

263

and I jokingly whispered to Manuel, "Just exactly what are we building here — a destination resort for international fugitives?" I was surprised at the sharp look that he tossed me, and at his lack of humor. Sitting beside me, Winfried looked surprised and concerned at what he had just heard from Otto.

Our last night in San José, Winfried called my room and said to come down to the bar, where everybody was having drinks before going on to dinner. There were two players I hadn't seen before who were locked in talk with Otto at the corner of the bar. Otto introduced them to me — one, a pale, effetely good-looking man in his mid-thirties who apologized for his wheezing and shortness of breath, and explained that he was having an asthma attack; the other — his "business associate" — a stunning, slender blond woman who talked business seriously, but whose every word carried a hint of sex, although with a very hard edge. Both were German.

Otto said, "Richard, this is the gentleman who telephoned, trying to find me, when you were staying at my house in Port Grimaud. Well, he's finally found me, although a bit late, I'm afraid."

"Yes," the asthmatic German cut in, "and if you had told me then where Otto was, we could have saved millions — *millions!*"

"Relax," Otto said. "Richard was only following instructions. You'll have to forgive my young friend, Richard. He isn't as sick as he sounds. He always gets an asthma attack when he encounters a little stress — anything from his telephone bill to losing a few million." And with a wan but worldly smile that shrugged off the loss of a great deal of money, Otto a.k.a. Pedro excused himself to talk to some other people and left me with his friends.

"What is all this about?" I asked the German.

"I'm the president of Otto's company — well, one of them," he said. "I've been looking for him all over Europe and North Africa since I talked to you, and I finally tracked him down here — for all the good it does.

"As you know, Otto's got some problems with the German government, and with some people elsewhere. I had to get some instructions from him and his power of attorney. People were moving to block his bank accounts all over Europe. If I'd been able to find him, I could have saved most of it; but now it's gone — millions!"

"You mean Otto's lost *all* of his money?"

The German looked at me as though I were an utter fool. "Of course not *all* of it; everything except what he's got in Switzerland and here."

I was too fascinated to care about discretion. "And how much is that?" I ventured.

"How the hell should I know?" the German choked through a rasping cough. "I doubt that Otto knows."

After dinner, I got Winfried's lawyer alone in the hotel bar. I had noticed that he drank too much and talked too much. He had spent most of his career as a bureaucratic tax lawyer in the German government, and now, suddenly finding himself at the center of Winfried's and Otto's world of intrigue, wealth, and high international finance, he was inclined after a few drinks to unburden himself freely.

"What exactly *is* Otto's problem in Germany?" I asked.

"Well, the major one is a tax fraud allegation. He was the promoter of a rather large issue of tax shelter investments that were sold to professional people in Europe — mainly doctors and dentists. The government has the idea that there was something wrong with the deal."

"What's the amount of the government's claim?" I asked.

"Forty million."

"Deutsche marks?"

"Dollars."

I swallowed hard.

"Oh, don't look so shocked," the onetime bureaucrat turned suave international lawyer said. "That really is a piddling amount, and I don't think the government can make a case."

Since I was to leave the next morning, Otto suggested that I fly back to Miami with his German associates in the Lear that they had chartered there. It was a welcome suggestion. Flying in an executive jet was thoroughly compatible with the way I was feeling about myself. It also would give me a chance to probe for some more information on Otto. And I could get a refund on my ticket for that leg of the trip.

The San José airport was short on fuel, so we had to tank up at Camun Cay. Shortly after the Lear zoomed up from the tiny island, I said, "Is it true that the German government's price on Otto is forty million?"

It had been a congenial trip until then. The blonde, who had been flashing a calf and half a thigh at me, uncrossed her legs and stared out the window. Otto's partner was hit with a sudden attack of asthma and spent the rest of the trip breathing deeply from an elaborate inhalation contraption. Not another word was spoken until we landed in Miami and I said, "Thanks for the ride," and they said, "Good-bye."

I spent the night at the Fountainbleau and caught an early flight to San Francisco. After nearly a week of nonstop meetings and cocktails and dinners, with the constant need to be onstage every waking hour, the flight was a fine relaxation. I spent a lot of the time with my eyes closed, not asleep, but thinking without stress. It would be fall soon, and before long another year would be over. I had accomplished much, but a lot remained to be done — quickly.

I wasn't overly concerned that Otto and Winfried had been elusive and noncommittal when I insisted that I had to have a better deal to get involved with them. There was no way that I was going to participate for a mere ten percent of the capital that I raised. The deal was too big, and I had a feeling that my services and value would end up being far greater than those of just a fund-raiser. In a few days, I had already made conceptual contributions that had changed some of their basic thinking. I was also convinced that Winfried was out of his depth, that his trust in Otto was innocently misplaced, and that his naïveté was being exploited. The deal looked legitimate, but I was sure that Otto wasn't. The time would come when an expanded role would be necessary, both to save the deal and to get Winfried's fat out of the fire. And I intended to get paid for it.

They hadn't jumped at my proposal of fifty thousand up front plus expenses, and a piece of the action in addition to the ten percent, but I was confident they would come around. And I was sure there would be a lot of money to share — particularly since their answers had been nervously unresponsive when I had pointed out that, in studying their financial-planning documents, of the twelve they intended to raise from investors I could only find five million going for plant expenditures.

Otto had promised that, while he wasn't willing to put up any front money right then, or talk about an expanded piece of the action yet, I could count on an arrangement down the line that would make me happy. And, confident of my powers, I was sure I could count on it. So I promised them that I would get to work on the project. And I promised myself that I would end up with a large piece of the venture.

It had been a year of major promises.

I had promised Yolaine that I would make us and her family rich; I had promised Michael that I would pay back the thirty thousand he had guaranteed; I had promised the bank that I would pay my debt off; and I had promised Greg that very soon I would pay him the several thousand dollars that I again owed him for his high-quality, mind-sharpening cocaine.

In the year ahead, as I went about my business of raising money for Teildras and Costa Rica, and for a life-style to match the visions, I knew, without a touch of fear, that I would have many more promises to keep.

7
Promoter

To be a successful promoter, you have to be effective in five dimensions. You have to have a captivating vision. You have to have a credible plan for making the vision real. You have to be articulate and persuasive. You have to look and act successful. And you have to be single-minded.

I had acquired all of those capacities. There wasn't anything I couldn't do. I had always been *intellectually* articulate and persuasive, but now, thoughts that in other days I would have had to reach for came with astonishing swiftness, and were expressed with a polished assurance that had the ring of undoubted success, as I became not only a brilliant advance planner of tomorrow's triumphs, but a master of their extemporaneous advocacy.

Cocaine gave me the courage of single-mindedness. Emboldened by the new powers I felt, I left behind my prosperous but mundane profession, overburdened with spirit-quenching details and dull people. I didn't bother to tell my clients. I simply quit working for them, and plunged headlong into my new life; a life freed from banalities and committed to the large ideas and bold concepts that I had become so good at.

Gone were the fears of my childhood, and the anxieties

and frustrations of my adult years. The man whose innate gifts and high promise had been crippled by years of gnawing insecurities had been put away. In his stead stood a man whose powers were to be respected, and whose words were to be trusted. I discovered that I was irresistible to many people, and certainly to myself. Cocaine had killed the fears and unleashed the power. I buried the past and became a promoter.

With the new challenges that I faced, with their relentless demands on my time, energy, and mental sharpness, cocaine became an essential companion for all my waking hours, which were becoming longer and longer, as the time allocated for sleep progressively shrank to accommodate the requirements of planning, promotion, and increasingly frequent late nights of intense conversations at the little French bistro. Without cocaine, I got tired very quickly, and I found that I couldn't think as fast. And the words didn't come as quickly, or with nearly as much wit. Without it, I felt that others found me less compelling; and, with my perception of their diminished response to my charm and will, flashes of the old insecurities would come. I no longer kidded myself that my stepped-up use was a temporary aberration. The truth was that I could no longer either play comfortably or work efficiently without cocaine. And I liked myself infinitely better with it. And that was that.

If my dreams were to come true, I needed to raise some money very fast. I had some cocaine, and drafted up an interim financing agreement for the Teildras project; it wasn't quite the same as the one I had used for Donald and Calvin, but some of my thinking had changed. Then I had some more cocaine and called my brother Bill, a newspaper editor in Salt Lake City. He was very impressed with my description of the property, and the profit I promised him, whether he just stayed in the deal for the minimum six months, or for the duration. And he had liked Yolaine a lot when he met her at my father's funeral. He bought a seven-thousand-dollar share, and got a lawyer, who was a close friend and trusted him, to put up another seven thousand. And I marveled at the convergence of circumstances that, after all the years of neglect, had brought me close to my family again, and I was glad that I could share my good fortune with them.

When I finally got all the papers together that were necessary to get Yolaine into the country, I flew to France. We had a few fine days with her parents at Teildras, then spent a few more in Paris, where we had a dinner at Maxim's and reminisced about our first date, another at Faucheron's, where we had first said we loved each other, and a lunch at Brasserie Lipp, for which we had no sentimental excuse, only a desire to spend a noontime at one of Paris's hottest spots. It was a great week; my fortunes had never looked brighter, and for the first time in quite a while I had enough cash to be able to spend it without nagging fears of the imminent future.

But, back in San Francisco, I realized that the cash was going to get perilously low sooner than I had expected. I had a lot of traveling to do — a trip to New York to talk to a financier about getting some money together for an investment in the Costa Rica project; a trip to Washington to confer with Commodity Credit Corporation people about the financing of soybean purchases, and to arrange with the Overseas Private Investment Corporation for insurance to protect my investors; and I was sure another trip to France would be necessary before long. Plus, I would be having a lot of large expenses for business entertainment right in San Francisco, and then there were Yolaine's and my own living expenses, and I needed to get the Porsche's engine rebuilt; it was burning oil and losing power.

I had some cocaine and drafted the first of my interim investment agreements for the Costa Rica project, which also permitted the investor to pull his money out in six months at fifty-percent profit. Then I had some more co-caine and telephoned my sister Mildred in Portland, and eloquently explained the project and what a good idea it would be for her and Joe if they had some surplus funds that they wanted to make a handsome return on. She called me back after conferring with her husband, and said that they were excited about the deal and appreciated the op-portunity, and if I would send them a copy of the agree-ment they would send me a check for thirteen thousand dollars. I explained that I couldn't hold the deal open for the time that would take, but I would fly to Portland in the morning to close the deal. I had a couple of large snorts on the airplane just before getting off to meet Joe in the Portland airport. They withdrew the money from a high-interest-bearing account that they kept for their retire-ment. And Joe told me how happy he was to be getting into this kind of deal with somebody he could trust, be-cause they had recently lost fifteen thousand dollars in-vesting in a real estate deal with a person who turned out to be a crook, and they couldn't afford to lose any more money. He was looking forward to retiring from his dental practice in a couple of years, and the profits from my venture would be a real help, and he felt particularly good because it was a no-risk situation. Although we seldom saw each other, I had always had a special soft spot in my heart for Mildred and Joe, and they for me; there had been an unspoken bond of understanding. I was especially glad that they could share in my good fortune.

A couple of months later my brother Bill called and said that his lawyer friend needed his money back for another investment. I didn't have the seven thousand and, more-over, for reasons I didn't understand, most of what I had had only "yesterday" was gone.

I hadn't planned to raise any more money for my Teil-dras project until I had an agreement with Le Comte, and there in fact *was* a project. But the costs of entrepreneurship were unexpectedly high, and it was necessary to move forward. Besides, I *knew* there would be a project, and I knew it would generate a fortune.

So I had some cocaine and drafted a new interim investment agreement for Teildras, a little different from the last one, to accommodate the different circumstances, and had ten copies made. My brother Tom met me at the Seattle airport. As he had promised on the telephone, he had arranged a meeting with a number of his fellow doctors at the clinic. Tom would buy a seven-thousand-dollar share and so would his son, and he was confident that, among his colleagues, another three shares could be sold to give me the thirty-five thousand that I had told him I needed. I was sure of it too. Doctors and dentists were always looking for deals, particularly if they involved real estate and had a tax shelter twist. Not only did my agreement promise them a lot of sheltered profit; it gave them an opportunity, if they stayed in the deal, to buy my condominiums in France at cost. The deal was irresistible and, jacked up with cocaine, so was I. I ended the day not with the thirty-five thousand I had been looking for, but with forty-nine. I was on a roll. Tom was one of the country's leading breeders of Arabian horses, but the costs of the operation had gotten too high, and he had decided to liquidate his stock at auction. He was impressed with all of the high finance I was involved in, and, at dinner, said that he had a beautiful big white three-year-old that would make a wonderful present for Yolaine. If I wanted to buy it for her, he would take it out of the auction and give me a good price. I looked at the horse, and he was stunning — sixteen hands, which was almost unheard of for an Arabian, with a royal tail set. I had always loved horses, and the animal would give Yolaine the thrill of her life. Then it occurred to me that it was stupid to have just one horse, so I added a second to the purchase order and made arrangements for my brother to ship them down to San Francisco after the first of the year.

The horses cost me ten thousand dollars, but I felt that they were a small extravagance that we deserved. I had, after all, been working very hard, and they would give Yolaine and me a wonderful hobby to share. I could still easily pay back Bill's lawyer friend, and have enough money left to do what I had to do to raise the really big investments that would be needed for Teildras and Costa Rica. But I would have to get cracking.

The transactions with Tom were particularly satisfying. Among all of the family, I had always felt that he was the most judgmental about my apostasy from the church, and my life-style in general. It was rewarding for me to see how impressed he was with my large business interests, and with the casual ease with which I had bought his horses. And he was pleased, too. He had taken great satisfaction when one of the doctors said, "Richard, your deal really looks great; but I'm sure you know that we're doing this because of our knowledge of Tom. Any brother of Tom Smart's is somebody we feel safe doing business with."

Just before Christmas, I raised fifteen thousand dollars on Costa Rica from a major San Francisco politician. I had worked a lot with him in my efforts to get federal funds into San Francisco. He had seen me work my magic in Washington, I was quietly supporting his political ambitions, and he had a world of confidence in me. When I called him to tell him what was on my mind, he invited me for a drink at the Olympic Club, gave the Costa Rica investment agreement a cursory glance, said, "It looks okay to me," and agreed to give me fifteen thousand. It didn't bother me at all when he said that he almost certainly would exercise his option to get his money back in sixty days with a twenty-percent profit, since he wasn't invest-

274

ing for the long term, but just wanted to give me the temporary help I needed. No problem.

I bought some cocaine to energize me for my third trip to New York in a month to chat with my financier friend about my projects, and the cost of my stay there was unexpectedly high. When I got back I bought Yolaine a thousand-dollar wristwatch for Christmas and wished that I could have gotten something better, but thought it prudent to conserve funds for the tasks ahead. On New Year's Eve, we gave a lavish black-tie dinner party for our six favorite couples in our new San Francisco apartment. It had been a good year for me and my friends, and I foresaw the new one as positively bullish. In celebration of the good life, I put thirteen hundred dollars' worth of cocaine on the table.

In January of 1981, Winfried telephoned me in much distress from Cologne. He said that there had been a big scandal in Germany involving the sale of tax shelter investments, with a lot of bad newspaper publicity. "Nothing related to our Costa Rica venture, you understand, but, in the present climate of investment mistrust, it will be impossible to sell our securities here. If the deal is going to go forward, all of the capital will have to be raised in the States."

Almost as an afterthought, he mentioned that Otto had been arrested at his Paris apartment, after surreptitiously coming into France on his Costa Rican passport to visit his wife. He was sitting in a Paris jail, fighting extradition to Germany.

Winfried's charismatic mentor, and the real quarterback of the Costa Rica venture, had been put away, and with no idea of how to proceed, Winfried was in a panic. He had a lot of money sunk in the project, and it had become obvious that he was financially strapped. We agreed that I would take over the principal role and get the lion's share of the deal. I would come to Cologne and we would re-structure the deal to be more responsive to the American investment market. Winfried agreed to my insistence on a payment of thirty thousand dollars upon my arrival, to cover my costs.

After our week in Cologne, and with Winfried's check in my pocket, Yolaine and I went to France to tell Le Comte and La Comtesse about the Teildras project, and give them the proposal. They were thrilled with it. In Paris, I had paid five hundred dollars to get the fifty-page document translated into French, and Le Comte, whom I felt suddenly at ease calling Papa, was thoroughly im-pressed with my business acumen and articulation. When Yolaine and her parents and I walked out into the street after dinner at an Anjou restaurant, Papa put his big arm around my shoulders and said, "Richard, I can't tell you how wonderful it is — what you are doing for the family."

I was more pleased with myself than I had ever been. The turn of events in my life had been at once strange and magically rewarding. Through my astuteness at busi-ness, of all things, I had been elevated to a new level of respect with my own family, and had won the love of my wife's. Astuteness and, yes, vision, generosity, and a deep well of goodwill.

8
Harvest Time

In 1976 I had sown the seeds of a new life. By 1981, from the once-barren fields of my past, lush new visions and happy realities had sprouted, fertilized by ever-more-generous doses of the glistening white powder that dissolved problems, embellished dreams, and made all things possible.

Nineteen eighty-two and -three were to be the season of my harvest. I had looked to gather sweet fruits, but a blight had infected the garden, and the crop had turned a withered, ugly brown. The dreams were dead and the fantasy life was finished. Success was not the task at hand; survival was.

In July of 1983, as Yolaine and I watched the last of our household goods being loaded into the moving van, I didn't know where 1982 had gone, or for that matter even '81 or '80. All I knew was that I had been constantly in motion and had realized too late that all the movement had been on a treadmill mistakenly thrown into reverse.

It was necessary to get out of town for a number of reasons. The most pressing one was that I had no future in San Francisco. Every day people were demanding their money back. The Teildras and Costa Rica projects were dead in the water. The glory path of drugs and illusion had led to the brink of an abyss. Nobody — not *anybody* — trusted me, I was living on cocaine, and I had forgotten how to earn a living.

But things would be different in Washington, D.C. There, away from the giddy environment of indulgence where I had lost my bearings, and removed from Greg and instant access to cocaine, I would cleanse my values and kick the drug. The three of us — Yolaine and I had an infant son now — could start a new life there, at the scene of so many early triumphs — the place where my name still evoked respect and where I had powerful friends in important places. I was sure it would be so.

Unlike Humpty Dumpty, the polished porcelain shell that was the façade of my San Francisco life didn't fall and crumble all at once. It went piece by piece. There had been some early chips on the surface that, if examined closely, would have warned of a structure too fragile to endure. But I had maintained my promotional gifts almost to the last, and had been able to divert the attention of all but the most keen-eyed from the signs that announced the beginning of the end.

Among the deceived, I was the most gullible of all. Even as the wounds widened, and health and honor flowed from me like rivers of blood from an unstanched hemorrhage, cocaine continued to fuel my powers of self-delusion.

Only my friend James saw clearly early on. Or at least he was the only one of my close friends who was willing then to face the painful truth of my forthcoming doom. In the early spring of 1982, James suggested that I vacate the space he had been renting me in his law offices in the Bank of America Building. I knew it was a hard thing for him to say. James and Catherine had become, with Michael and Alice, my dearest friends. For over a decade we had skied together, vacationed together, dined and wined and laughed together. We had agonized as parents together, as we watched our children grow into adolescents and then adults. It had been Catherine who had cared so much that I find a good woman to fill the void left by a broken marriage, and it had been James who, late on a crisp June night that seemed so long ago, had in tipsy merriment introduced Yolaine and me in a French kitchen, and it had been the two of them who first feted our fresh love at their home and who, with caring, had monitored the progress of our love ever since. James and Catherine had been at the core of our life.

It wasn't just that I was months behind in the ridiculously low rent I was paying James. Despite his skepticism, he had wanted to give me some support in my new entrepreneurial ventures, and had been charging me only six hundred dollars a month for the space *and* the use of a secretary, *and* a telephone. No, it wasn't the rent problem at all. What James said was, "Richard, it just isn't working out." People I owed money to were calling all day long looking for me; and, even though I wasn't connected with the law firm, people didn't make that distinction, and he couldn't have the firm's reputation tarnished. Also, he had a number of young lawyers recently out of school whom he was trying to impress with the need for disciplined work, and my work style wasn't a good example. He didn't mention that my hours had been completely unpredictable, that the secretary could never tell anybody where I was or when I would return, and that for weeks papers had been piling up on my desk in great heaps, disorderly and unlooked at. And, although he didn't say anything about it, I knew that he thought my behavior had become erratic, and that he was troubled because he didn't know how to approach me about what he thought was a problem. Alone among my friends, James didn't use coke, so *of course* he had trouble communicating, and, despite his goodwill, we had grown increasingly apart. James cared a lot about me, but his consciousness hadn't been elevated and he lacked the gift of special visions.

Fortunately, Greg came up with an idea to solve my office problem. He had recently gotten closer with his first wife — the straight one whom I hadn't met yet — and he was helping out with the sale of her house and the details of her impending bankruptcy. He said that she had once had a blue-chip advertising and public relations firm on Montgomery Street, but had fallen on hard times. She was rebuilding her career, had a nice little office out in the Potrero district, and I could use space there free of charge.

The "office" turned out to be a renovated garage that had once had a tiny apartment over it, and it was decorated with a seedy red carpet and metal desks, but I was grateful to have it. I couldn't very well invite business people over, but I had a telephone and could get letters typed. A few weeks later, Greg said that he was moving his coke business into the office. His neighbor had put a shotgun under his chin and told him he was going to blow his head off if he didn't close down, so that all the crazies would quit showing up at all hours of the night.

Greg had been in the office only a few days when he started introducing me to everybody as his partner in the Costa Rica project. He had become very fascinated with the venture and wanted to contribute a lot of ideas. And he wanted some share of the profits, since we were sharing everything else. I guess he had a right. He had wired me six thousand dollars in France when I had needed it, and had financed a trip to Costa Rica with money he borrowed from his girlfriend, and I now owed him close to fifteen thousand dollars for cocaine. I didn't mind Greg's unilateral assumption that we now were engaged in a common, lifelong business relationship; it was his *telling* everybody about it. His sheepskin jacket, and the sickly pallor and drug-dulled eyes, announced a world far removed from the pinstripes and brisk countenances of Montgomery Street, where, high up in gleaming towers, I had so recently plied my entrepreneurial trade. I had a difficult enough time explaining why I had moved my office. Now, I had to worry about a new balancing act — keeping close enough to Greg to take advantage of his cocaine and small emergency loans and moral support in times of crisis, yet keeping far enough removed to ensure that my upscale friends and business associates wouldn't figure out the depth of our connection. Greg simply was not their type; nor, for that matter, was he really mine. Or so I kept telling myself.

All of Greg's old Sausalito crowd — the former wives and girlfriends, and sometime carpenters and unemployed housepainters, Tommy the Thief — now hung out in my office, getting sage advice from Greg, and buying and snorting cocaine. And there was an assortment of new characters, the most ubiquitous of whom was Phil, the gynecologist employed by a big pre-paid medical service company. He surreptitiously moonlighted for the proprietors of an infamous and frequently raided sex theater, giving the girls their periodic VD checks and presumably doing an occasional abortion. Greg rented Phil the office at night for his moonlighting medical practice. It was a good deal for Greg; he not only got a little rent money, but also sold Phil a lot of coke. He bought a lot to pass on to the girls, and the doctor himself was a hard-core addict.

Greg's ex-wife number one, the official tenant who was struggling to reestablish a respectable little business, was at first beside herself with confusion over the endless stream of characters flowing in and out of the office. But Greg assured her that some were consulting clients he was advising and others were people with whom he was involved in "ventures"; "some big deals were going to come down soon in addition to the Costa Rica project," and he was going to have a lot of money to help her with her problems. She smiled wanly, puzzled by the appearance and manner of all these entrepreneurs, but happy that they were part of Greg's plan to restore her good fortune.

No, I couldn't figure out where those years went and how they vanished so fast. In the last few months of 1979 and the first few of 1980, when the visions were fresh, I had established my talents as a promoter. And that was good, because ever-larger amounts of money had to be raised in the next couple of years. I never did get around to raising the real capital necessary to develop the Teildras and Costa Rica projects. God knows, I tried. But the problems kept popping up — legal problems to resolve and technical details to work out and paperwork to be done and nitpicking questions to be answered ("Well, what about the problems next door in Nicaragua; won't they endanger the investment?" — petty questions like that). All the kinds of mundane, boring, spirit-suffocating activities and attention to detail that engaged bureaucratic minds, but were anathema to a brain that had been liberated from dross for a destiny of visions and great ideas made real.

But until such time as I could get the petty details of the big ideas taken care of, which would enable me to go after the required millions, I had to keep going after more "interim" financing. "Interim" financing was the money needed for more "planning." And for more talking. And for more traveling. And for supporting me and my wife and my baby while I was planning and talking and traveling. There was so much *movement* in those years, and so much money was needed to finance the movement.

There were three trips to Costa Rica, three more to Paris and another to Cologne, and repeated journeys across the continent to New York and Washington and back. I couldn't stop traveling — to have meetings and to plan and to raise more money. Always, more money. The demands of my own support were heavy. Yolaine and I had to try, as best we could, to maintain the life-style that was essential to the image of a successful promoter and his wife. The horses alone were costing five hundred a month to board at a suitably exclusive equestrian club. And, as more and more early investors demanded their money back, "interim" financing took on an expanded meaning to include new amounts that had to be raised to pay off old obligations. And the new amounts were much larger than the older ones, because of the large short-term profits I had promised in order to get the early money.

My life became one of perpetual motion. Motion to get new money to pay off old money. And travel took on a rationale of its own. Sitting still, the festering problems threatened to suffocate me. In the motion of travel, I felt the rush of success. To *move* from place to place was to evade the doubters and elude the vultures and to get closer to the consummation of the vision. And still more motion to get more and more cocaine to ease the stress and fuel all the other motion necessary to bring dreams to fruition and reap the harvest. All was motion; nothing was rooted in a solid, stationary place.

One morning in late 1981, I picked up the *San Francisco Chronicle* and read a story about a confidence man who had ripped off people in Beverly Hills for millions of dollars and then disappeared. The story said that the con was a classic Ponzi scheme. I had never heard of Ponzi or his scheme. Apparently Mr. Ponzi was the one who made an art form of the discovery that you could quickly get vast amounts of money by capitalizing on other people's greed. All you had to do was invent a grandiose project, however thinly documented, for investors. And the more grandiose the better; paradoxically, grandiosity always seemed more credible to the greedy than simplicity. And you promised everybody a tremendous profit for a very short term investment. Then, when those obligations were coming due, you would go to other investors to get money to pay off the first investors. And, with your credibility established, and all your original investors happy with the money you had made for them, you could go back to them for some more, and to still newer people who had heard of your success. The problem was that, eventually, as the total obligation got bigger and bigger, you ran out of investment sources, and the game was up because there never had been real earnings to pay anybody with from *any* projects. Indeed, there were no projects. A Ponzi scheme, the article said, was a crime.

I was struck for a moment with a shock of recognition; if people didn't understand my motives and the *ultimate* reality of my projects, what I had done superficially looked very much like a Ponzi scheme. My obligations had climbed to well over two hundred thousand dollars and I had no immediate way to meet them. But I certainly was no criminal. I hadn't intended to do anything like *that*. And my projects *would* succeed. They *had* to succeed. Yolaine and I had our dreams. They were *real* projects, not con jobs. Didn't my projects exist in my head, and on hundreds of sheets of paper designed and refined and eloquently articulated through countless inspired nights? Of *course* they did! No problem. Everything would work out. And, besides, I had a deeply felt *moral* obligation to pay back my family and friends, whatever happened to the projects. I threw the paper into the trash can and had a large helping of cocaine to prepare myself for the new day's fund-raising.

One beautiful Sunday in May of 1982, Yolaine and I went out to the equestrian club to see our horses and have a picnic. Yolaine was seven months pregnant, so she couldn't ride. I went on a short trail ride on her big white horse and he was especially happy and spirited that day. After the ride I met Yolaine at the picnic area. I had been a little tired, so I had privately had some cocaine, and the drug confirmed that I shouldn't be bothered by the irksome detail of taking the horse back to the stable. Instead, contrary to one of the basic rules of horsemanship, I tied him to a flimsy picnic table. In a few minutes, a brisk wind came across the meadow and, surprised, he reared, and then ran off down the road, dragging the table. I ran after him, and when I got to the stable area I saw a group of people clustered around the horse. Terrified by the table bouncing at the end of his halter rope, he had run up an embankment and had fallen between two parked cars, and had torn his right foreleg out of its knee socket. He was standing on three legs, and his other one was hanging by a few exposed bloody tendons; he had to be destroyed. I wouldn't let Yolaine see him because of the pregnancy.

The death of the big white horse seemed an omen to Yolaine. When I had given him to her, she had told me of her recurrent dream of a big white horse when she was a little girl, and had said that my surprise gift to her was a profound symbol of my romantic fulfillment of her dreams. A symbol of grace and loyalty and courage and truth.

Yolaine wept in bed that night, and said that the death of her white dream horse symbolized the collapse of our lives and the death of our goodness. I told her that I shared her sadness, but that she shouldn't generalize a tragic melodrama from one unhappy event. I had tried to keep most of the bad news from her. It had been months since I had started unplugging the two phones from their jacks, leaving just enough of the prongs inserted so they looked operational. But when our friends kept telling her that they could never reach us because there was no answer, she had found that ruse out. And much of her time had been spent plugging phones in after I had unplugged them, even though I had promised her I wouldn't. And she had learned too much of the truth about the sources of the money that I still managed to bring in, the magnitude of our festering debt, the bankruptcy of my dreams, and the gathering of the barking jackals who would not be denied their share of the carcass.

I loved her with all my heart, and convinced myself that the lies which had become a habit were to protect her and our unborn child from grief. Not just the lies about money, but about cocaine. The instant she had found out that she was pregnant, she had given up everything that was bad for the baby — even tobacco and caffeine — and she asked me to promise that I would cut down on my cocaine use. She had enjoyed it a lot herself but, even before the pregnancy, hadn't used it habitually, and she had grown increasingly worried about my dependency.

Mel, the friend who had introduced me to the drug, had spent over a week in a coma after an attempted suicide, and as soon as his recovery was assured, Nina had left him to live with a twenty-year-old surfer in Hawaii.

Congressman X had a ruined political career and a shattered life. At one public hearing, his nose had started spouting blood. At another, he had flown into an uncontrolled, rambling rage at a witness, filling the air with a torrent of obscenities. His wife had left him, and during his almost weekly trips to California, he had repeatedly ignored scheduled meetings with his staff and his constituents, and, feigning illness, had locked himself for days in a room at a Howard Johnson's, accompanied only by stale, half-eaten hamburgers and piles of cocaine. His affliction had become an open secret, and he had been forced to abandon any thought of reelection and go into therapy.

And almost daily Yolaine read in the press of deaths and lives ruined. She had complained of my growing testiness, and had worried aloud about the failing health that she thought she saw written in the lines on my face and in the heavyweight bags below my eyes. I assured her that it was only temporary fatigue and stress, but she begged me to cut down, and I lied that I already had — "Now-

adays, sweetheart, it's only an occasional social toot" —
when, in truth, I was using cocaine at my desk like coffee,
from morning until midnight.

On July 24, 1982, Geoffrey was born. Yolaine had taken
wonderful care of herself and the pregnancy had been
uneventful. The doctor said that she was in perfect health,
and was built ideally for childbirth. We had purposely
conceived Geoffrey at a time when I was at the top of the
roller coaster, and life looked very good. But even with
our fortunes in a temporary slide, the expectation of a
baby had brought Yolaine and me closer than we had ever
been, and we looked forward to the birth with eager love.
Despite the mounting troubles, I had managed to persuade
Yolaine that everything really was coming together and,
in her resilient trust in me, she was confident that I would
recoup. Our child would be a privileged one, given the
best education that money could buy, and raised in dignity
and honor.

Yolaine was two weeks past due when, on a Saturday
afternoon, she began having abdominal pains, and her skin
got cold and clammy. I managed to reach our obstetrician,
and he said that, while it didn't sound like labor, I should
take her to the hospital and have the obstetrics nurse ex-
amine her. The nurse took one look at her and rushed her
onto the table, and attached the fetal monitor. In less than
one minute the room was full of rushing people, and the
nurse told me that the baby was distressed, with a greatly
reduced heartbeat, and that an emergency cesarean was
necessary. With an intravenous contraption already stuck
in her, they wheeled Yolaine into surgery.

Only twenty minutes later, the nurse returned and told
me that I had a baby boy. Our obstetrician arrived only
in time to close the incision, and he told me that what had
happened was a miracle — impossible. In twenty minutes,
Yolaine had been prepared for surgery and anesthetized
and the surgery had been completed — by a twenty-six-

year-old Vietnamese woman, who was the resident surgeon on duty. He said that he didn't know anybody with twenty years of experience who could have accomplished that. The placenta had started to break away from the uterus prior to labor, and Geoffrey's oxygen had been seriously reduced, and further delay in the birth would have meant either death or brain damage. The way the doctor put it was, "Another ten minutes and, at best, the baby would have been dead. And your wife was in danger as well. She's lost a great deal of blood, but both she and the baby are fine."

I wept with relief and love. And I was glad that Yolaine didn't know of the position that I was in. The cost of the crisis would turn out to be six thousand dollars, but I had let our health insurance lapse and couldn't pay the hospital a dime. I had two hundred dollars in my pocket that I had borrowed from Greg, and three hundred dollars' worth of cocaine.

Yolaine was badly anemic from blood loss. The doctor said they could give her transfusions, which always carried some risk, or she could resign herself to several weeks of inactivity and go on heavy doses of iron. We decided on the iron, and she stayed in the hospital for ten days, with instructions to spend another couple of weeks largely off her feet at home.

About a week after I brought Yolaine and Geoffrey home from the hospital, I woke up in the middle of the night with a strange feeling of liquid on my face and the taste of salt in my mouth. I got quietly out of bed so as not to wake Yolaine and went into the bathroom and turned on the light over the mirror. My face was covered with a sticky red liquid that already was congealing in my beard, and a thick steady stream was flowing from my nose. I hadn't had a nosebleed since I was a child. The image of my haggard, bloodstained face cut through the stupor of my half-sleep and stared at me like a ghastly apparition from Hell.

There seemed to be an awful lot of blood, and I was frightened. I lay down on the bathroom floor and plugged my nostril with toilet paper and pinched the top of my nose between my fingers. It took a long time to stop the hemorrhage, and by the time I did, every towel in the bathroom was soaked with blood. I stayed on the floor for a long time and calmed down. I reminded myself that one's own blood is a frightful thing to see, and it always looks as if there is more of it than there really is.

In the morning, I told Yolaine what had happened and said that she shouldn't be frightened when she went into the bathroom. "I'm fine now," I said, "and I'm sure it won't happen again. And, remember, it always looks like there's more blood than there really is." We both knew it was the cocaine, but neither of us said anything about it. I had told her that I had cut way down, and she didn't want to call me a liar, and, most of all, she was worried about my health.

The hemorrhaging continued on and off for four days, usually in the afternoons when I was in the office, and in the middle of the nights. But despite Yolaine's pleading, I refused to see a doctor, assuring her after each attack that I was sure it would be the last one. I didn't want to do any more damage to my nose, so, for a while, I would insert the straw under my tongue, where there were exposed mucous membranes for quick absorption, and would suck the coke up that way.

One day, after an especially severe hemorrhage at the office, I came home to go to bed. After about an hour there, I felt very strange, so I took my own pulse. It was a hundred and twenty-eight, and I told Yolaine that I had decided to see a doctor. I called Phil, the cocaine-addict gynecologist, told him what the problem was, and asked him if he could arrange for me to see somebody at his hospital. He said that I should be careful with the coke for a while. "There are other ways of taking it," he said. "Have you tried it under the tongue?" I told him that I had already figured that out, but I was grateful for his medical advice.

While in the hospital waiting room, I nearly passed out. The doctor said that a small artery at the top of the nose — "what we call a shooter" — had broken. He tried to cauterize it, but the lesion was too big, so he packed it. He said that I had lost three to four pints of blood. I had to stay on the table for six hours, taking liquid intravenously and getting my blood pressure back in order. The doctor said that the attacks had left me anemic and gave me a choice between transfusions and iron tablets. I opted for the iron, and spent most of the next week in bed. Greg gave me some more coke and some money for groceries.

Two days before Christmas that year, I got a letter from an attorney representing several of the investors in my Teildras project. The lawyer said that he had reviewed the investment agreement, with all my assurances of no risk and large profits, and all of the correspondence I had sent over the months explaining delays and problems. He said that he had concluded that I had violated state and federal securities laws and that, unless I made immediate arrangements for repayment, he intended to file a civil lawsuit and also refer the matter to the county attorney for prosecution.

I asked my attorney, Al, the Montgomery Street lawyer whom I had met at Greg's and who now dropped by the office every day to snort coke with us, to reply for me. Although Al had his own problems — his wife, along with Greg's girlfriend, had gone into the hospital for six weeks of drug therapy, and his thirty-thousand-dollar BMW had been repossessed and the mortgage on his four-hundred-thousand-dollar house foreclosed — he was very helpful.

His letter pointed out that the lawyer's "investigation," which had led him to conclude that I had assets and a life-style indicative of available money, was erroneous, since my own Porsche had been repossessed and I had been threatened with eviction for nonpayment of rent. The lawyer agreed to await receipt of a long-term repayment plan.

In the spring of 1983, my brother Tom telephoned me and told me that he had paid all of the doctors the money that I owed them. He was a man to whom personal honor was everything, and he felt responsible; the act was typical of him. But, while that was a relief from an immediate threat, it was only a small dent in the larger catastrophe.

After I had repaid Calvin's first small investment, I had gone back to him for a larger one. I owed him twenty thousand, and he wanted his money.

Donald had increased his investment to twenty thousand, and he wanted his money.

After I had repaid the politician's first small investment, he and his law partner had given me another thirty thousand, and they wanted it.

I had gotten a prominent San Francisco architect and friend, whom I had retained on speculation to do the Teildras project design, to invest thirty thousand in Costa Rica, and he wanted it.

I had gotten twenty-five thousand from an old law school classmate and, unable to repay it, I had assigned my share of my father's estate to him, and my family was unhappy about the complications that had caused, not to mention their own uncompensated heavy investments.

And I had gotten thirty-five thousand dollars from my college roommate, who, in my younger years, had been my closest friend in all the world; and now, with his anxious phone calls unreturned, the lawyer he had retained was making it plain that, unless I repaid him, he would reluctantly have to sue me.

Yolaine's father had needed thirty thousand dollars to

reduce the debt on Teildras, and I had sent him a check, confident that I could raise the funds during the month it would take for the check to clear from Europe. But I hadn't been able to get the money and the check had bounced, ruining his credit, which until then, though it had been marginal, had always been honorable.

And I had been summoned to the office of the California Franchise Tax Board in a criminal investigation of my failure to file tax returns. When I had appeared for the interview, I had been stunned and frightened when they read me my rights and had me talk into a tape recorder. It was true that I hadn't filed state or federal tax returns since the year that I first started using cocaine, but I had *intended* to. I wasn't a tax-evader. I *respected* the government. I wanted to *be* in government. It was just that the difficulties always got in the way, and I had always planned to file a little bit later. Besides, I was sure I didn't owe that much; I hadn't really worked for several years, and all the money I had turned over was for business expenses, wasn't it? Or at least most of it. My lawyer worked out arrangements with the state and federal tax people, but there were still a lot of details to be addressed. And I couldn't find a lot of documentation. I didn't *have* any documentation. For years, details had bored me, while I had focused on the large concepts that would change my life. In fact, ever since I had abandoned my consulting practice and gone to Lake Tahoe with a cocaine-raised consciousness and a book to write, I had found it impossible to fill out *any* kind of forms, or even answer routine mail, let alone fill out tax returns. For all those years, uncompleted forms had grown in stacks on my desk, then gotten stuffed into drawers — along with even older yellowing papers and age-faded envelopes containing messages of things to be taken care of "tomorrow." Somewhere, as my consciousness had soared toward the stratosphere, leaving behind the mundane occupations and enervating details that constricted ordinary mortals, it had become an immense emotional challenge to face any kind of bureaucratic task. With my brain churning up a firestorm of creativity, I could turn out in a day fifty pages of captivating analysis and rhetoric for one of my projects. But I was emotionally incapable of even getting my driver's license renewed.

A three-thousand-dollar check that I had given the Cariari Hotel on Yolaine's and my last trip to Costa Rica had bounced. I had been sure that I could cover it before it got to my bank. But I hadn't been able to.

It wasn't that I hadn't tried to get new "investments" to take care of all these matters. In the last months before the collapse, I had, in desperation, called everybody I could think of. I called Tom Brokaw — after all, he had just been promoted to national news anchorman at a salary of over a million — and asked him for eighty thousand. He was sympathetic, but he couldn't do it. I called old law school classmates, some of whom I hadn't talked to in twenty years. Joseph Hetzel, who I thought had family money and was now teaching law in Cleveland. Adam Walinsky, who had brought me into the Kennedy campaign and was now a rich lawyer in New York. Dave Jones, a pioneer in for-profit hospitals, who had founded Humana Corporation, whose sales that year had exceeded two billion. I had even made a fast trip to New York and met with, among others, Peter Tufo, who had been John Lindsay's man in Washington, and had later been successful in law and been engaged to Lee Radziwill. They were all glad to hear from me, and had all, as graciously as possible, let it be known that they thought I was crazy.

A lot of the people I called from San Francisco in those last days, with "an investment opportunity so profitable you can't possibly turn it down," thought it strange when I told them there was no number where they could call me back after they gave my offer some thought, because

I was calling from a phone booth, but "don't worry about it, I'll call you again myself in an hour." As the crisis continued to deepen, it hadn't been enough just to unplug my phones at home at night. Now, I was afraid to spend too much time even in the remote and forlorn garage/office where Greg sold coke and I conjured and promoted elegant business deals. The place had working telephones that were answered by a lazy, quasi-Chinese person of uncertain sex whom Greg's first ex-wife had hired for pocket money to pass for a secretary, but who lacked both the initiative and imagination to give me credible protection from the insistently pursuing telephones that afflicted me everywhere, demanding money.

So I made the lobby of the St. Francis Hotel my part-time office, placing dozens of calls from its telephone booths and charging them to the "office" number, then going back to the velvet divan in the lobby bar to order another martini, and then finally to the restroom to fortify my courage for my follow-up phone calls with another couple of quick hits of coke. None of those phone calls in the blurry twilight of my entrepreneurial career paid off — the promoter's bright brass sheen had gone green-black with tarnish — but the St. Francis was a shelter that afforded a kind of comfort in those terminal days. Until one early afternoon when, after countless fruitless phone calls and too many martinis, I fell asleep on the velvet divan and then — how many hours later? — felt a strong hand gently shaking me by the shoulder. The St. Francis's assistant manager asked me if I was a guest at the hotel, and I slurred back that I wasn't but I loved the ambience of the place, and he asked me to please leave and not come back. He apparently was new on the job and didn't realize that I was a person who, only a year or so before, in a silk tuxedo, had attended an exclusive and very swell dinner dance after the film festival in that very same hotel and had danced with Goldie Hawn and had kissed Mayor Feinstein on the cheek.

It was the same afternoon that the sole of one of my Gucci loafers had started to separate from the upper leather, which was worse than unfortunate since the loafers were the last pair of shoes I had, not counting my Adidas running shoes, which were still in good condition because I didn't run anymore. I walked out of the St. Francis without umbrage or any other feeling of any kind whatever, and found my way to a shoe repair shop. Despite the piles upon piles of unrepaired shoes with pale yellow identification tags affixed to their laces, I convinced the happy Greek that it was essential he put my crippled Gucci at the front of the line and immediately reattach the sole to the upper because I had a meeting with the mayor. With a skeptical "oh sure" kind of chuckle and with pride in his work, he accommodated me and I gave him a bad check for sixteen dollars.

The carnival was over, the lights of the dream were burning dim, and everywhere darkness gathered. I felt a shapeless mass of nerves rubbed raw, soft flesh bloated by the gin and bourbon I constantly needed to smooth out the coke jangle, glassy eyes, and a brain that floated everywhere and yet was nowhere. The cocaine had quit working the way it was supposed to. I wasn't golden anymore.

The last six months in San Francisco, I lived in a haze of cocaine and liquor. I don't know exactly when it happened — sometime during my last futile Costa Rica trip, I think — but cocaine's effect on me suddenly changed. Or, if the change had been occurring gradually, I hadn't been aware of it. The first time I sensed that something was very different was in the bar of the Cariari Hotel. I had been negotiating for three tough days with a Nicaraguan for the sale of the industrial contract I had been awarded by the Costa Rica government, and the negotiations hadn't gone well. After dinner, I had gone to the restroom to stoke myself with a huge dose of cocaine, and then returned to resume the talks. I got the usual energy rush and the flood of fluency, but none of the euphoria that had been my drug's best gift. And there was no new beauty; the bar still looked tacky.

Back in San Francisco, it became much the same — a couple of snorts would give me the critical lift, but without the magic. It was common knowledge that a lot of heavy coke users often suffered deep, crippling depressions when they came down from the drug, but I had never been one of them. It was true that, as my use had gotten heavier in the last year, I had experienced some minor letdowns when I was off the drug, but nothing serious. Besides, the times when I wasn't wired had become so few that the question of postdrug depression was really academic.

But now a strange thing was happening. I felt a kind of depression even when I was *on* the drug, which was nearly all the time. Not a *crippling* depression; a shadow of disquiet and despair that constantly lurked below the surface of my energy and restless movement. The coke still made me *believe* in the reality of hopeless fantasies, and allowed me to ignore harsh truths. But it was a belief without joy, and I became aware of enemies. Whatever was going wrong was other people's fault. I could still tell jokes and, with the help of coke, occasionally break through the darkening clouds to raise Yolaine's spirits and entertain friends with a dose of high humor, but more and more I became edgy and lived in a state of subdued testiness even when fully wired.

I needed coke in the morning before breakfast and all day and all evening long. And to keep the wired edginess in check, I needed alcohol all day and all evening with it. There weren't many emotional ups and downs those last hazy months, because I was wired and semidrunk all the time. I moved about on a flat plain, accompanied everywhere by futility. But that dark companion was made palatable by cocaine's still active power to clothe even the bleakest reality in a fetching and diverting costume — even though now, when the light and shadows were just right, I thought I occasionally caught a fleeting glimpse, beneath a disguise that had grown threadbare in places, of ugliness revealed. But when that happened, I would have some more coke and some more liquor, and then some more of each, and soon the view would get reassuring again, if not as surpassingly beautiful as it once had been, when my drug was new.

The coke sustained the lies and, as always, helped them look noble. In that, the drug hadn't lost any of its felicity, and that was good because the intricate, delicate structure of lies — and it was a structure to which I added a new support almost daily — had become the foundation that carried my very existence. Lies to myself and to everybody else. It was imperative that I keep the structure erect, now adding a strut here, then a beam there — an endless construction of an edifice to fantasy that had no finish. To end the building process would be to court collapse and disaster. But as long as I could keep buttressing here and reinforcing there, the edifice would remain standing, despite its increasingly grotesque shape.

From the very beginning, that had been one of cocaine's great qualities — it made it clear that, whatever my purposes, whatever my strategies, and whatever my words, they were *good*. They were good because they were *mine*. The truth was what I said it was, and where there *were* discrepancies, cocaine had made me confident that eventually my powers would make reality conform to my view of it.

With my life in rapid decay, the psychological sanction that cocaine gave to the lie was as compelling as ever, but employed toward very different ends. The game wasn't promotion and triumph anymore, but evasion and survival; yet the drug proved as facile in putting a face of imagined decency on clear corruption as it had been, when the light was rosier, in disguising soaring fantasy as serious and responsible business. Now, the bad checks weren't to finance transatlantic flights and settle extravagant hotel bills. Instead, they went to the grocer and to the nice butcher on the corner just so we could eat, and to the long-suffering landlord, who finally got one too many returned unpaid and told us to get out. And now, the elaborate, eloquent, impassioned presentations weren't for the purpose of romancing excited investors into surrendering their money. Instead, they were to calm the nervous and pacify the outraged — to persuade the betrayed that their money was safe and their trust deserved, as would all become clear "in just a few days," when first this imaginary event happened, and then that one.

The drug had gone sour, but in its power to make me *believe*, it was constant. The bad checks were okay, because tomorrow something good would happen and I would cover them. The lies were okay, because the projects *would* happen, and eventually would make everybody whole. The lies were mere details and necessary, and they were redeemed by a larger purpose that was *good*. Even though I was on cocaine most of the time, I knew there was a difference between other people's reality and mine; but I also knew that reconciliation of the discrepancy would occur when the world moved to share *my* line of vision, which was where truth was.

Once cocaine had been a recreational wonder, a handmaiden for fanciful, fun trips of the imagination. With a little bit of heavier use over a little bit of time, it had become a wonderful stimulant for my intellect and a help in creative business. With addiction and a failed life, it became the killer of conscience, the black angel that accompanied me everywhere, assuring me that death was life, that wild churnings of a disoriented brain were wisdom and enlightenment, and that corruption was honor misunderstood.

The last weeks in San Francisco, I felt my personality slipping away. I spent a lot of time walking around the neighborhood feeling vacuous, like a spiny epidermis-shell that still moved, even though empty of the sea animal that had been its life. I would explain to all the merchants in the Laurel Village Shopping Center how the checks they had gotten back had been caused by a bank mistake that soon would be rectified; and others I warned in advance of checks that probably would be coming back because of the big mistake, and they acted as if they appreciated my dropping by. When I wasn't doing that, I often went into the Sugar Plum bar to drink bourbon and read the newspaper while waiting for something to happen that would change my fortunes. Most of the time, I wore my blue stretch-material jogging suit with the white stripes, and if I met friends who asked me what I was doing in the neighborhood in the middle of the day, I told them I had been jogging. I had the feeling that nobody believed me — not the grocer nor butcher nor drugstore clerk nor bartender nor any of the acquaintances I saw on the street — and that, when they looked at me, they didn't really see me. At home, when I looked in the mirror, I saw a person with sunken eyes and sallow skin who had turned fat, not pleasant to look at and probably worse to talk to for very long, and I understood why others' vision fogged over and their words went hollow at my approach.

Sometimes at night, if I had enough to drink and Greg's coke was of decent quality, I could feel my personality come back. Well, I wasn't sure it was the same one I had had, but at least it was *a* personality, and for a while I would feel less empty. I would pack my nose with coke and then I could talk briefly with the old conviction, but more often with the new testiness, to Yolaine; and then, in grotesque imitation of an earlier life when a dream was fresh and a spirit was innocent and vital, I would make urgent and articulate phone calls to no particular purpose until dawn. The euphoria that once had been cocaine's blessing never came back, and the old charm showed itself in only rare and fleeting glimpses, and then with a bitter edge. But refueled, the lies would resume their quick and easy flow, and when they did I felt an identity again.

But hardly anybody had a use for that identity anymore, not in any of its guises. I had betrayed my family and friends, and except for my daughters and my baby boy and Yolaine, who somehow had retained her faith and strength, I was quite alone.

I had to get out of town. Away from failures. Away from the haunting ghosts of years of "well-meant" lies. Away from the urgent clawings of an impending and very real doom. And most of all, away from cocaine. Self-delusion was ubiquitous, but even when deepest in its throes I knew that something was wrong. The lady had betrayed me.

In Washington, I would rebuild my life. I still had a large fund of prestige from the triumphs of earlier years, and it was time to draw on it. Alan Cranston had announced his presidential candidacy, and I was sure that my old boss would remember how invaluable my advice on issues and my speechwriting had been in getting him elected to the Senate. As a presidential candidate, Alan was a long shot. But he had been able to raise a fair amount of early money, had put together a crackerjack campaign management team, and, much to the pundits' surprise, was winning nearly all of the early straw votes in state party conventions, based on his single-issue campaign for a nuclear freeze and disarmament. The straw votes were only nonbinding "beauty contests" and didn't necessarily reflect long-term campaign strength, but Cranston's show of organizational strength had Mondale, Glenn, and the other candidates worried.

Hooking myself back up with Cranston seemed an astute way to get out of the pit and back into the mainstream of respectable life. I had met with Alan's sister, Eleanor, who adored me from earlier times, and told her that I wanted to write Cranston's campaign speeches, and she said she was thrilled. She had me meet with Alan and he was encouraging, but told me I should talk to the campaign management people. Greg and I flew down to a thousand-dollar-a-plate fund-raising dinner at the Beverly Hills Hotel. Eleanor had arranged for me to get in for free so I could meet with the press secretary. Greg gave me some coke so I could get myself ready, and the press secretary was impressed but noncommittal, and said he would be in touch.

That was good enough for me. Although I was determined to get off cocaine, the time was not quite yet; and, during that period of dislocation and change, it was good to have the coke still in my brain to help make reality appear better than it was. For my wife and friends and the people to whom I owed money, I had a pathological need to put an angelic face on the devil that was more intense than ever. So, I returned to San Francisco and had a good jolt of coke, and told Yolaine and my friends that I had been hired as Cranston's speechwriter. It wasn't *really* a lie. I was absolutely full of confidence. For the first time in months, with the cocaine there had come an intimation of the old feeling of power. Eleanor and Alan and the press secretary had all *sounded* enthusiastic; sure — I as good as had a commitment. Once in Washington — *actually on the scene* — my credentials and well-known talent would carry the day — and Alan and I would formalize the deal. I was sure of it.

I had some more coke before meeting with Calvin to ask him for another four thousand dollars to finance my moving costs. I told him about the wonderful new job that awaited me in Washington, and convinced him that the additional money was needed to protect the large investment he already had in me. Over drinks in the Great Electric Underground in the basement of the elegant Bank of America Building, I consummated the last of my successful "promotions." I wouldn't be in that kind of building again for many years, if ever. The kind of building where large deals are made by men of means and good reputation.

My conscience wasn't offended by these lies to my wife and my friends, for they were necessary to get me on my way to Washington, where, quickly, the world would come right.

I couldn't get a job in Washington, and Yolaine and Geoffrey and I lived in the Washington Holiday Inn for nearly two months, spending all the money that we had planned to use to pay the movers when they delivered our furniture, plus the little bit of cushion that we had planned to live on until my first paycheck came in.

The first few weeks, I walked almost every morning over to the Cranston headquarters to talk to the top staff people about my job. The first few times we had serious talks and they would say something like, "Touch base with us tomorrow." Then they started saying, "Give us a call next week." And finally the receptionist would tell me that so-and-so "isn't available right now, but you're free to wait." And I waited a few times for a couple of hours and then, when nobody ever appeared, left to find a bar for a morning drink. And then, when I left the hotel in the morning, instead of going to the mythical meetings that I told Yolaine I had scheduled with the Cranston people, I started going directly to the seedy little bar around the corner from the *Post*, where I had discovered that I could get martinis at ten in the morning.

I placed a dozen calls to Congressman Y, who had been

so enchanted by Yolaine and me at dinner, and who had been such a good friend over the years. None of them were returned, although when I went to his office his secretary did give me a handwritten note from him — a nice personal touch — that said he regretted that he couldn't be of any help.

I had breakfast with Barbara Boxer, who had been an old colleague and was now a congresswoman from Marin County, and asked her if she had a good relationship with a local banker from whom I could borrow some money. She didn't say so, but I knew she was disconcerted by my appearance and manner, and breakfast with her was an embarrassment.

Yolaine and I looked at houses, as I assured her that the Cranston contract was about to come through, even though I knew it was dead. I was off cocaine. The coke was out of my blood and brain, but it had left its mark. I still couldn't face reality, and the habit of escapist lying that the coke had made so easy died hard, even long after the drug was gone.

I called up my old and good friend from the Kennedy days Sally Quinn, who had married *Washington Post* editor Ben Bradlee, and tried to borrow six thousand dollars; she was gracious and glad to hear from me, but she couldn't do anything.

I wrote a letter to my old college fraternity brother Bill Marriott, who had inherited the Marriott hotel empire, asking for a job in his legal department. He had his executive vice-president and general counsel, who also was our fraternity brother, call me and ask me out to the offices for a talk. Sterling was friendly but said there wasn't anything.

I didn't know whether the word had gotten out on me, or whether it was the way I looked and acted, but it was clear that in Washington — the town where I had been a young star not so many years before — I was dead.

One night I met an articulate black hustler in the bar of the Holiday Inn, where, in lieu of cocaine, I had been drinking a lot. He ran a small foundation dedicated to teaching poor black people how to run cooperative businesses; and, impressed with my background, he offered me a job writing proposals for a few hundred dollars a month. And I went to work in the bowels of Washington's poverty-infested ghetto.

It was enough to live on, but not enough to support my wife and son. I called Ron, my former partner in San Francisco, whom Yolaine and I had entertained in a Madison Hotel suite with caviar and champagne when she first came with me to Washington. Although I already owed him twelve thousand dollars, he came over to the Holiday Inn and loaned me another six thousand dollars to pay for Yolaine and Geoffrey to go back to France to live with her family until I could get something going, and to pay the hotel bill, and to give me a little to survive on until I had money coming in. For security, I gave him the diamond ring that I had had made from Yolaine's mother's antique earring at the time of our marriage.

My black friend provided me a small apartment with a mattress on the floor, a table and two chairs, and many cockroaches.

Yolaine and Geoffrey stayed with me for two days and nights before they left to live with her family in France. Yolaine and I slept on the single bed–sized mattress, and Geoffrey slept in a borrowed crib. They were two strange and painful days, in which Yolaine and I held hands a lot and embraced with our cheeks together, but said very little. It was as though we both had unconsciously set ourselves against feeling with too much intensity the reality of what was happening. If we talked too much about it, emotions would come untethered and our walls of stoic resolve would crumble. So we loved each other quietly as the hours passed away, each of us alone in our thoughts.

304

On our last morning, Yolaine took me by the hand and said, "Richard, I love you with all my heart and I always will. I'm not leaving because I want to, but because I have to. We have a son and we can't raise him with this daily uncertainty. You do understand, don't you? *Please* understand, my dearest."

I told my wife that I understood.

"And, darling," she said, "I know we'll be together again. I *know* it with all my heart. You'll get yourself strong again — oh, *please*, get yourself strong. And you'll get a good job again, and we can have a wonderful life together. We still can, you know; we really can. I don't have to be rich, you know, I never really did care about that. All I need is security and a good life for my son. That's *all*, my love. That, and honor. Promise me that you'll do what you have to, to get me and your son back with you. *Promise* me."

And I promised her that I would.

We rode on the airport bus to Dulles pretty much in silence. We checked the luggage in and got Yolaine's seat assignment, and had a drink in the lounge. Pan Am announced its Paris flight, and Yolaine walked with Geoffrey in her arms to the door of the boarding bus. At the entrance she turned around and smiled with tears glistening in her eyes, and Geoffrey waved. He was just over one year old.

Afterword

I THINK it is virtually impossible for an addict to be cured, even with the best professional help, unless he can truly believe that he still has something to lose. Where there is a belief that everything worthy in life has already been lost, the reservoir of motivation is drained dry. At the nadir of his life, the addict must have somebody to affirm his dim hope that — with job, money, friends, and self-respect gone — there remains a source of caring, a source of potential validation of his worth as a human being. I was lucky to have Yolaine and Geoffrey to give me clear signals that, however degraded my life had become, they wanted me — indeed, needed me — and would be there for me if I merited trust. And the message that they would not be there if I stayed on the same course was as important as the declaration of love itself. The healing of a drug addict is commonly thought to require compassion from others. In fact it requires them to be tough with the addict as well. He must know that he still has something cherished to lose; but they must also let him know to a moral certainty that, without recovery, he will in fact lose them.

Yolaine, Geoffrey, and I are reunited as a family. I am cured of my cocaine addiction and know that there will not be a relapse. The three of us enjoy excellent health. We cherish each other in a way that is possible only for those who have consciously known and overcome an immediate threat of total loss. Just *being* has become a fact of great importance. I pass each day with an acute awareness of the fragility of life, savoring unremarkable hours that, in younger years, I would have taken for granted.

There was no single turnaround point that came to me in a flash of enlightenment. I didn't have the benefit of suddenly being "born again," of suddenly feeling cleansed of sin, clear of eye, and transfigured into a strong being of instant righteousness. All my life I had wished for something akin to Paul's instant revelation of truth on the road to Damascus; but it didn't come in the years when I was trying for it, and it certainly wasn't about to come in the years of relentless decay. The realization of impending doom, and the desperate desire for rescue, grew step by step, as I sensed that I was approaching the bottom of the ladder into the pit.

My friends James and Catherine gave me a clear message of their love, and of their disgust. Their tolerance had run out; they wouldn't be manipulated anymore, but they would be there if and when I could live truthfully. My brothers, whom I had relieved of large sums of "investment" funds at the height of my drug fantasies, made their outrage plain; but when I finally mustered the strength to confess the addiction and the lies that germinated in its depths, they offered forgiveness and renewed love — provided I worked to redeem my life. My sister told me: "You don't need anyone else's forgiveness. You only need to forgive yourself." That was both the gentlest and the harshest statement of them all — and the truest.

The explicit statements of friends and family — the unvarnished condemnations of what I had done to them, emotionally as well as financially — were vital. As long as there was a suggestion of continued tolerance among people I cared about, I would continue on the path of deceiving them and myself. But now I was hearing that the game was up and all avenues of further illusory escape were closed. That message and the message of love — not sentimental love but tough, hard-edged love — were essential ingredients in my marshaling the will for recovery. I had been thrown a lifeline. If I was going to get out of the pit I'd have to climb the rope with my own strength.

I found part of that strength in retrieval of memories of long lost years that, however anxious, had been honorable and rewarding. Reaching consciously into my past to retrieve what was good, I tried to make it live again as a psychic ingredient that would substitute for drug fantasies. But a large part of the strength — the operational, resolute strength — I got from my wife. From Yolaine came the daily energy I needed for my search for the scattered pieces of my former self, and the moral glue to paste a life back together.

In honesty, I don't know what would have happened if Geoffrey had not been born right at the time when I was fast sinking to the bottom. It is quite possible that I would have finished the fatal plunge and, exploiting Yolaine's gifts of love and loyalty, taken her with me. Or she might have left me to save herself, drawing upon her reserves of self-respect and her unquenchable thirst for a life in the sunlight. Ours was a storybook love affair, but no more immune to life's disciplines than any other.

But Geoffrey *was* born and I think his birth was a large part of our salvation. Even though I was still in the grasp of addiction, the appearance of fresh, unsullied life, utterly dependent on his parents for a decent chance of fruition, was a sobering event. I was proud of him and I loved him and I was a drug addict — although my now unambiguous condition was not something that I or anybody else had yet openly acknowledged. I wanted my son to be proud of his father and to grow up with a decent chance for the best that life had to offer. I was the most adoring father who ever lived, yet I knew I was immobilized.

Yolaine was different. If there's anything fiercer in purpose than a loyal wife and passionate lover, it's a woman who has given birth to a child. For too long she had been vulnerable to my deceptions, but she never had a talent for deceiving herself.

When our love was new she had been swept away by my charm, saw me as a hero, and trusted me implicitly in all things. Despite her initial misgivings, it had been easy to seduce her into joining me in my cocaine pleasures. As I immersed her in my life of affluence and indulgence, she came to relish cocaine as a marvelous entitlement of the privileged elite — something to be careful with, but certainly not a threatening evil.

With her pregnancy, she had quit the drug immediately. And then, with a new son barely delivered, she discovered the poverty, the lies, the hundreds of thousands of dollars of debt. Briefly, she sank into despair, but it turned quickly into outrage, and then into a resolute strength.

She demanded to know why I had hidden the truth from her. Lamely, I explained that I had wanted to protect her from distress in her pregnancy. Infuriated by that implicit condescension, she asked why, if that was so, I had continued to lie after the birth and was, in fact, still lying every day. I didn't have an answer.

She joined the ranks of disaffected siblings and friends. She was not going to run off at once with Geoffrey to the château and parental security — that would be too easy. She was going to love me, encourage me, and if necessary bludgeon me into health, and into rediscovery of the worthy person who, she assured me, she knew still existed. But if that failed she eventually would leave; she had no other choice. Suddenly I was no longer her mentor, but a chastened student. And a young woman, not quite thirty, was my teacher.

Yolaine's ultimatum did not work an immediate miracle. I continued to take cocaine for many months, and after that liquor became a problem. And even with the cocaine finally out of my brain, the habits it had fertilized had a residual stamina: For a long time I couldn't quit lying to put a rosy face on a black reality. But Yolaine persevered, and her courage gradually nourished my own.

Above all, she demanded the truth. Whatever yesterday's lies had been, she could handle the truth — however terrible it was — if I could just tell it to her *today*. And, bit by bit, I discovered that facing reality, however bleak, was less painful and exhausting than the relentless effort to hide it. It took a long time.

Truth was the most important idea. But Yolaine also spent her intelligence and energy in devising supports that, however prosaic they sound in the telling, were vital to recovered health. She taught me yoga, and I discovered that deep breathing and stretching, and a little unpretentious meditation, could make me feel wonderfully relaxed and good.

She cajoled and bullied me into taking up running again, which had been a long-forsaken passion. And I discovered that an urge for a snort of coke or a pint of whiskey could be quickly dispelled by some strenuous exercise. If there was an element of self-flagellation in that (and on many occasions I did punish myself beyond prudence), there also was a wonderful sense of elation at the accomplishment.

Yolaine knew it was impossible to be a meditator and a runner for very long and still be a drug addict and a drunk. It had to be one or the other; the body couldn't tolerate both. Her persistence made the choice increasingly easy. Every morning at five she rousted me out of bed and did an hour of yoga with me, then went on her run while I stayed with Geoffrey. She returned to push me out the door for my own exercise while she made breakfast before rushing off to her ten-hour work day at the public relations job that kept us alive during my long jobless months in Washington. Our living situation often depressed us. Our house was utterly barren of furniture except for a borrowed kitchen table and four chairs, because we could not afford to get our furniture out of storage. For a year we slept on the floor on plastic air mattresses with borrowed bedding, and we cooked in borrowed pots and pans. But the depressions passed quickly, cured by exercise and a rediscovered sense of humor. After all, wasn't our barren house a pleasant relief from the clutter of an overfurnished château? We had the advantage of a lot of living space, and there was nothing that had to be dusted or polished. As my body got healthier so did my spirit, and gradually I came to believe in possibilities again.

And she got me into church. Yolaine had had her problems with French Catholicism, and despite the goodness of the Mormon people, I had long since found their theology unpalatable. But we were both believers, I in my casual, nonworshiping, God-taken-for-granted way, and she with her peculiar personal amalgam of Catholic orthodoxy and Buddhism that — despite my teasing her about its hopeless theological contradictions — she had continued to practice, not in a church but in the sanctity of her bedroom, where I would sometimes find her silently praying for us in a posture of Eastern meditation while holding a rosary.

There was a Presbyterian church right next door to our Capitol Hill house. After many Sundays of watching worshipers going into church and hearing their hymns, Yolaine suggested that it might do us some good to join them. After a few more weeks of her careful prodding, we did.

It was a small congregation of warm people. Whatever else he said in his sermon, the minister opened each Sunday with the joyous announcement that "God loves you. Whatever you may have done, you can't destroy God's love for you. You're stuck with it." I had recoiled from much of what I'd heard in churches in my younger years, but that was a message that struck a responsive chord and I suddenly believed it. After the first service we attended we joined everybody in the Fellowship Hall for the coffee hour, and I was surprised to find myself easily saying, when somebody asked me what I did, that I was recovering from a cocaine addiction.

For a year, Yolaine's and my struggle had been almost entirely a private one; in the midst of vibrant Washington, we had lived in emotional isolation. Now, venturing into a church, freely announcing my past, and actively participating in the society of decent people became vital therapy.

Yolaine told me that she wanted to be a Presbyterian. I asked her if she intended to renounce her Catholicism and give up her Buddhist beliefs. "Absolutely not," she said. "I have no problem at all in being all three." For my part, I was simply grateful for the company of unpretentious, caring people engaged in a communal spiritual search. I had found that a place dedicated to elevation of the spirit wasn't a bad place for my reentry into the world.

I cannot guarantee that this recitation of the steps in my recovery is the best prescription for everybody who is trying to cope with a drug addiction, but for me it worked. I was blessed with one advantage that a lot of others don't have: a gifted and resolute person who was at once lover, partner, friend, and trainer. Miraculously, we have found that our romance, tempered into toughness by a searing ordeal, has flourished with a new vitality.

All that I have just said may sound like the classic happy ending. That would be a false reading. The aftermath of my drug addiction — even with the emotional and physical rewards of a detoxified brain and body — is an unrelieved struggle. The unraveling of the ugly consequences of my drugged years looks to be a difficult and lifelong task.

I had thought that kicking the cocaine monkey off my back would mean the end of my biggest troubles. It was a terrible thing to discover that ridding myself of the drug was only the first step in an arduous journey back to health, financial responsibility, and self-respect. The rebuilding of a life has been infinitely harder than was its dismantling.

Even with reconstruction of my own life well under way and with confidence in the future, there remains the enormous damage done to others. Even if full restitution were possible, the emotional wounds of betrayal remain. Betrayed trust heals with painful slowness, if at all, and the wounds of the innocent and trusting are the worst legacy of cocaine addiction.

The sudden popularity of cocaine that has occurred in this country since the midseventies is principally an upper-middle- and upper-class phenomenon. The drug's devotees are concentrated in a thin slice of society; many of them are in various ways influential and, in large part, they are engaged in professional, entertainment, business, intellectual, and political occupations. In the last couple of years, the greatly expanded supply of cocaine and its lower cost have made the drug increasingly a favored plaything of blue-collar workers and the middle-class young; but even with cocaine's "democratization" in the marketplace, it has retained its cachet as the drug of choice of the rich liberal establishment.

Any drug that offers an illusion of fast escape from overwhelming problems will appeal to the unstable, whatever their background and socioeconomic class. The mystery of cocaine is why *this* particular drug has seduced so many otherwise responsible, hardworking, outwardly successful Americans who, in earlier years, have not comprised a drug-vulnerable population (alcohol abuse is a *very* different order of problem).

The people who manage our businesses, give us our legal advice, run our banks, shape our opinions through the media, set our public policies through their votes in national and state legislatures — these are the kinds of people who, in only a decade, have become the most serious abusers in the greatest relative numbers of America's potentially most destructive drug. Why that should be so is one of the most important questions confronting our society. I believe my six years of experience with cocaine — first as my euphoric recreation and then as the handmaiden to my self-destruction — have given me some insights that help answer that question.

All of the cocaine users in the tight little circle of friends that I've described in this book — the millionaire investor, the international investment banker, the congressmen, the advertising executive, the drug dealer/law student, and myself — shared some basic characteristics. We were highly educated, prosperous, full of desire for achievement and recognition, and, above all, dominated by a concern for our public images. That profile, by itself, certainly isn't a prescription for cocaine addiction; it describes millions of Americans who have never touched an illicit drug and never will. But when you take that description and add to it another element — profound inner self-doubt — you have a person vulnerable to the seduction of cocaine and prone to eventual addiction.

From my own experience, I know that there are a few well-integrated people who are secure within themselves, whose inner realities coincide with the images they present to the world, who can use cocaine recreationally in a controlled way without great personal damage. (Why they would care to use it is another question.) In this book, Michael and his wife, Alice, were such people. Cocaine brought some problems into their lives that they could have done without; but they have been able to use the drug in a measured way for years without any kind of serious damage that is obvious to others, and certainly without the catastrophic consequences that it brought to my life. But they are the *only* regular users I know who have escaped relatively unscathed. For everybody else, the drug has meant erosion of dignity, severe damage, and despair.

For people driven by a need for success — or, more precisely, by a need for the *image* of success — and who compulsively pose as something that, in their own hearts, they truly doubt — for such people, cocaine is a set trap. It is the perfect drug to assuage the guilt and fear that, for many, accompany the climb to success; it enables fear to masquerade as high adventure; it aids and abets the extinction of that nagging moral conscience which is an uncomfortable companion to high ambitions imperfectly understood.

Talented people who are unsure that their inner qualities measure up to the external achievements that they believe the world expects of them become preoccupied with the conjuring of images to match those fancied expectations. And the more they become aware of their own image-making, the more they doubt their own authenticity — *regardless* of the fact that their objective contributions to their families, their constituencies, and the world may be meritorious indeed. For these people, driven to succeed but uncertain not only of their worth but even of their identity, cocaine does wonderful things. It reconciles their self-image with their idea of what they are supposed to be. For the first time, the cocaine user feels that he is everything he is supposed to be. For a while.

Cocaine gives the reticent the gift of eloquent speech; it makes the closed person open; it makes the uncertain feel infallible; and it makes the sexually insecure feel like erotic titans. The feeling of euphoria that cocaine induces is a consequence of the illusion of power. And for the individual who is preoccupied with a sense of powerlessness, however unconsciously, the temptation to repeat the experience is virtually irresistible.

In the early years of the current cocaine fashion, a lot of nonsense was written about cocaine not being "addictive," as that term conventionally had been used. Apologists for the drug announced that, while it might pose a danger for "unstable" people, it probably was a relatively benign recreation for most. Now, with cocaine indicted by a decade of devastated lives, psychoses, overdose deaths, and suicides, many experts suddenly have changed their tune and warn of the dangers.

The argument over whether cocaine is physically addictive or not has always been beside the point. For the great majority of cocaine users, the process of gradually increasing dependency that I've described does *not* involve physical addiction as the term has been traditionally understood; the cocaine user can be removed from the drug without going through the physical pain associated with withdrawal from a conventionally addictive drug. He may experience depression, irritability, or other emotional unpleasantness; but, when the drug has been ingested by inhalation, there is little evidence that it creates a "need" for the drug in the body.

That fact distinguishes cocaine from other hard drugs, but it is a distinction without a mitigating difference. The psychological dependency is at least as compelling — and is far more difficult to treat — than a physical addiction, for which medical treatments exist. It is far harder to cure a dependency rooted solely in the ambiguities of a disordered psyche. The habituated cocaine user is neither luckier, morally "better," nor easier to treat than the hard-core heroin "addict" whom society regards with emotions ranging from patronizing sympathy to outright contempt. In fact, the cocaine user may be worse off on all scores, notwithstanding society's present tendency to regard him, at worst, as a person with a minor and transitory problem and, at best, as a somewhat glamorous adventurer traveling in the fast lane of life. And whatever the drug's impact on individuals, cocaine may prove for society the most damaging drug this country has experienced.

If that last statement seems exaggerated, let me justify it. The human and social costs of cocaine abuse — in terms of illness, death, financial catastrophe, and shattered families — have become too well documented for even the most cavalier of the drug's apologists to ignore. But behind these terrible consequences exists the darker fact that, although not readily apparent, is both the cause of the obvious tragedies and a subtle agent of social decay in ways and places unforeseen: Cocaine fertilizes lies and nourishes the growth of liars.

That is the drug's alpha and omega. Whatever pleasures its advocates advertise, and whatever dangers its opponents warn against, the central fact about cocaine, and its frightening evil, is that it makes lies plausible, then acceptable, even pleasurable, and ultimately ubiquitous.

Heroin addicts lie, alcoholics lie, probably addicts of all stripes — whatever their particular drug pleasure — lie. *But it is not the same kind of lying.* The cocaine addict doesn't lie just to escape detection, or to find the means to buy more of his drug; he lies because he is riding a power rush that *gives him a right to lie.* The drug dissolves his insecurities, his doubts, his guilts; and, with repeated use, it also dissolves his conscience.

Most of us need the nagging of conscience. There are a few of us to whom one hundred percent honesty and virtue is as natural as a reflex. For the rest we rely on the discomfort provided by the inner voice; it is a mechanism we barely understand, but we know it prevents us from cutting too many corners and keeps us responsible to others and to ourselves. Cocaine destroys that mechanism.

About a year after I had kicked my cocaine addiction, I met with Dr. William Pollin, the director of the National Institute for Drug Abuse, to discuss the book I wanted to write. During our long talk about my experience, he wanted to know if I could describe what it was that cocaine had done to me psychologically. I had given a lot of thought to how the drug had destroyed my life in obvious ways, but, oddly, I hadn't ever put that key question to myself that precisely; yet, the answer came to me in a flash, starkly clear.

"Cocaine totally killed my conscience," I said. "I had never considered myself a thoroughly honest person. But before cocaine, I was always able to check myself before doing anything outrageously out-of-line; I always cared about honor, and I generally was able to keep within the bounds of common decency. After I got deeply into cocaine, there *were* no bounds. It wasn't that I didn't know when I was lying, but that I felt I could lie with moral impunity. I was specially endowed and specially empowered; I was embarked on great causes, and the ends totally justified the means. My conscience was simply dead."

Dr. Pollin's expression told me that was an answer he had not heard before, and that it had struck a chord of recognition. His reply was short — "The death of the superego." What he said struck me less than how he said it — a near whisper that communicated both discovery and concern.

Psychiatrists call it the superego, we laymen call it conscience, but it all comes to the same thing. It is what makes us reasonably ethical and moral and caring, it is what enables us to live together in society. And cocaine utterly destroys it.

The danger posed by this aspect of the drug is particularly grave for two reasons.

First, cocaine does not obviously disable most of its users for a very long time. To the contrary, its effect on many

318

people is to make them feel more competent, and indeed *appear* more competent to those they are dealing with. They believe in themselves more, become more eloquent, and lie with absolute credibility. Cocaine's erosion of the public personality can be a subtle and slow process, and the addict's practice of deception can be extraordinarily effective for a very long time — indeed, right up to the very threshold of the inevitable collapse. By then the list of victims of the wreckage — people who in various ways have been duped — usually includes many beyond the addict's family.

Second, the composition of cocaine's premier constituency — outwardly "successful" people who lay claim to rights of leadership and who influence values — raises a frightening spectre: Unless cocaine use is effectively curtailed, or suddenly goes out of fashion, the circle of "victims" whose lives are adversely affected, however indirectly, by drug-induced deaths of conscience will expand to include us all.

There is a truth to be told about cocaine and its devotees among America's privileged, however harsh and elitist it may sound in the telling: When something that is a vice in grimy alleyways becomes a fashion openly indulged in the parlors of a socioeconomic-political establishment, the very foundations of society are at risk. Drug abuse among society's certified failures is a profound unhappiness for the individual victims; a cocaine epidemic among our establishment could become a practical calamity for the country. Individual illnesses and social illness feed on each other.

My friends and I shared an emotional disorder — the wide gap between our ideas of success and the public images we manufactured, on the one hand, and our profound inner securities and self-doubts on the other. That disorder is hardly unique to cocaine addicts. Such inner conflicts have long been a major concern of psychotherapy.

319

But in our particular time, changes in our society have transformed a manageable disorder into malignancy.

I have referred to the impact of the sixties upon my life and the lives of my friends. Two things happened in this watershed decade that relate to the severity of the emotional disorder afflicting many of my generation, and our affection for cocaine specifically. In a rush of enthusiasm for new enlightenments and revolutionary politics, traditional values were tossed aside. Then, the psychologically sustaining social causes that replaced those values were shattered. In the vacuum, the so-called New Morality flourished.

The life I've described in this book was ripe for seduction by the New Morality in general and cocaine in particular. It is not only my life; in outline, it is the life of the many people in America's privileged, success-oriented class who have adopted cocaine and its attendant licentiousness as central elements of their life-styles. It is the life of the outwardly brave and internally fearful.

This is what distinguishes my generation — a generation that I would describe as comprised of people roughly between the ages of forty and fifty-five. Many more of us have the unhappy emotional profiles than previous generations had — and if our relative numbers are no greater then it is demonstrably true that we have not been as capable as previous generations of managing our emotional afflictions. We have plunged into escapist, negative behavior at a rate and of a magnitude unprecedented in our society.

A year or so ago, social commentators prematurely predicted the passing of the cocaine "fad." The drug was going out of fashion, they said. They were lethally wrong. The traffic has increased enormously and has spread through all segments of society. Like marijuana before it, cocaine has moved out of the dark corners where "far out" social rebels indulged in it, into the center of the lives of millions of "straight," mainstream people. At the height of its fashion, the worst that could be said of marijuana was that it benumbed the brains of a lot of people a little of the time, and of a few people nearly all of the time; and turned the very few who made a life-style out of the herb into lifelong daydreamers and welfare cases. But cocaine is addicting millions with euphoric illusions of power made of false realities; and slowly, subtly, and perniciously it is undermining the traditional social ethos, and psychologically sanctioning behaviors whose touchstones are selfishness, inconstancy, lying, and betrayal.

By now it is clear that stepped-up law enforcement isn't going to solve, or even make a visible dent in, America's cocaine problem. The evil is less in the drug than in ourselves. Ultimately it's a matter of values. Through self-knowledge we must try to accept who we are; and if, in knowing ourselves, we find that we are unacceptable, we have to try to change — not through drug-abetted escapism, but through confrontation, humility, and hard work. We must try to know and accept the society we live in; and if, in knowing it, we cannot accept what it has become, we have to try to change society as well — not by using drugs to make reality appear to be something other than what it is, but by working to shape good new values to replace the old ones that we have carelessly abandoned.

Cocaine is not just another drug. It is the perfect expression and symbol of a society that, behind a robust façade, is rootless, drifting, and in search of a fix.